Mastering
the Curved Blade

MASTERING THE CURVED BLADE

Steve Tarani

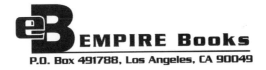

EMPIRE Books

P.O. Box 491788, Los Angeles, CA 90049

First published in 2008 by Empire Books

First edition

08 07 06 05 04 03 02 01 00 99 1 3 5 7 9 10 8 6 4 2

Printed in the United States of America.

Empire Books
P.O. Box 491788
Los Angeles, CA 90049

Library of Congress Cataloging-in-Publication Data

Tarani, Steve,
  Mastering the curved blade / by Steve Tarani. -- 1st ed.
     p. cm.
  Includes index.
  ISBN 978-1-933901-40-4 (pbk. : alk. paper)
  1. Knife fighting--Training. 2. Self-defense. I. Title.
  GV1150.7.T367 2008
  613.6'6--dc22

2007052662

CONTENTS

PART II—PERSONAL SAFETY

PART III—DEFENSIVE TACTICS

INTRODUCTION

Since the mid-1990s my full-time occupation has been that of both small arms and defensive tactics instructor. A subsection of my responsibilities falls under the category of knives—that is safe usage and personal protection.

Predominantly in the area of defensive tactics, a knife is considered a close-quarters personal defense option. It has been quite a struggle, to say the least, for law abiding citizens to exercise their constitutional right to own and carry firearms for personal defense. It's amazing to me that law makers continue to serve their own political agendas and try and pass more and more legislation to limit the means for law abiding citizens to exercise such a fundamental constitutional right as the Second Amendment.

Following the media blitz of unfortunate criminal incidents, the liberal, anti-constitutional left repeatedly aids the sick and twisted momentum of "criminals don't obey the law and criminals have guns so let's place more gun restrictions on law abiding citizens" illogic.

Somehow we, as law-abiding citizens of a free republic, granted certain inalienable rights by the Constitution of the United States of America, have bought into this media-induced erosion of the Second Amendment, that which the founding fathers of this great nation saw fit to place second only to freedom of speech—a right that was paid for in blood and the ultimate honorable sacrifice: the lives of our ancestors.

It's a terrible shame that we as Americans are rapidly following in the footsteps of other nations such as Great Britain and Australia. Both of these countries have completely stripped their citizenry of all rights to personal defense with a firearm. Today, law abiding citizens of one of these nations are forced by their own government to sit at home with the doors and windows locked in abject fear as looters, rapists and murderers freely pick and choose their victims knowing full well that there's no chance of being confronted by a firearm. Do we really want that to happen here in the US?

Given this rather unfortunate state of affairs it remains incumbent upon the citizenry of this still-free republic to call upon our voting powers and reach out to communicate our thoughts and our opinions to our state and federal representatives regarding this critical matter. We as Americans have the right to own and carry firearms—plain and simple. There's no complex language involved.

Unfortunately some of us reside in near-communist bloc states that place extreme restrictions on firearm ownership—defying the US Constitution and challenging the very fiber of our personal rights and freedom as Americans. Criminals still get to own and carry firearms, but thanks to legislation, we the law abiding citizenry are forced to give up this right on their behalf. Personally it's very disturbing and without a doubt Washington, Jefferson, Adams, Franklin and other founding fathers, must spin around in their graves when they see the atrocities that modern vote chasing legislators inflict upon our constitutional rights with regards to defilement of the Second Amendment.

Given the unfortunate state of affairs listed above, this manuscript is intended as a supplementary guide to personal defense options by means other than a firearm, and more specifically with the use of a curved blade. If your particular operational environment—at work, home or while traveling abroad—prohibits the carry of a firearm, then a knife is the very next best problem solving tool. The curved blade is an especially good choice, as it has certain personal safety and defense advantages over the straight edge knife.

As this remains an unclassified (public) document and is therefore available to bad guys as well as those of us on the right side of the law, all *offensive* techniques and methods have been carefully and purposefully omitted. What remains is a fully functional and comprehensive overview of the usage and development of both personal defense and safety skills with the curved blade.

Following publication of my first book on the karambit (an Indonesian version of the curved blade) back in the late 1990s, various knife makers augmented the curved blade market resulting in today's wider variety of models from which to choose. If you compare what was available in 1998 to what's available today, the number of curved blades for sale has increased substantially. Given the increase in interest as well as more curved blade owners, more and more questions have sprung up over the years regarding selection and usage of the curved blade. It is from these numerous inquiries over the past decade or so from which this manuscript is born.

The training material contained herein is intended for the law-abiding, defense-minded, first-time owner of a curved blade who may possess little or no background in the usage of curved blades (or straight blades—or any personal safety training whatsoever), as well as those who have had some prior training in this area. For those of us concerned about our own personal safety and the safety of our loved ones, who have an open mind to develop additional skills and a willingness to absorb useful information, this volume is full of valuable training technology.

The information contained herein is designed to provide familiarization and working knowledge of the curved blade as a problem-solving tool in the event of an urgent need for personal safety.

PART I
THE FUNDAMENTALS

A BRIEF HISTORY

The roots of the curved blade stem back centuries and accounts vary based upon cultural perspective. Relying on minimal written record and a predominantly oral history, it is difficult to pinpoint the exact origins of the curved blade. It has been estimated by my masters (senior-level edged weapon instructors hailing from Malaysia, Indonesia and the Philippine Islands) that the curved blade goes back before the Common Era.

In ancient times, the larger two-handed sword version of the curved blade—called a klurit (sometimes spelled "clurit" and pronounced "klee-ur-eet") preceded the handheld, personal version of the curved blade by generations. Originally called a "karambit," a name still used today, the smaller handheld version of the curved blade was very similar in development as the dagger was to the English broadsword, the dirk to the basket-hilt sword of Scotland, and the wakazashi to the Japanese katana. Essentially it was the companion tool to the ancient Southeast Asian villager. But how did these curved tools end up in America? The same way the Scottish dirk, the English dagger, the Spanish daga and the Italian stiletto did—it traveled with the folks who immigrated to America.

We are most fortunate to have trained with the torch bearers of the arts that utilize the curved blade: devoted and skilled teachers such as Guro Dan Inosanto, Sulaiman Sharif and Guru Besar Herman Suwanda. These instructors have preserved this knowledge and background for future generations. Only as a result of the masters' willingness to share these arcane skills and through extensive training am I am able to pass this valuable information directly on to the reader.

Although rumored to have been brought to America around the late 1800s (which is very possible), the curved blade was "officially" introduced to the United States sometime in the late 1950s and made popular, especially via the martial arts community, through the late 1970s and 80s. Virtually unknown in the secular community, by the mid-1990s it was predominantly recognized as a utility tool and martial arts training implement derived from the heritage of Indonesian Pencak Silat, Malaysian Bursilat and Filipino Kali.

The predominant use of the curved blade in ancient times was originally similar to the uses of the European utility knife. Field work like cutting twine or rope, chopping fruit and vegetables, digging holes, scoring leather, and was found in some rare cases to be an exceptional personal safety blade. Through constant refining of this unique tool and its usage, the ancient villagers of West Java found it to be a superior utility blade and to possess a distinct advantage over other knives in the event of close quarter combat. Thus, these early villagers adopted the curved blade as part of their daily accoutrement and introduced it into their indigenous hand-to-hand combat survival systems. The curved blade caught on and was adopted by inhabitants of neighboring villages and subsequently those of surrounding islands. The Indonesian warriors of old embraced the curved blade as their edged utility tool and last line of personal defense.

In recent years, researchers of edged tools (and their usage) have identified the curved blade as the premier utility blade of the ancient Javanese village dweller due to its versatile functionality. Things haven't changed all that much over the centuries. The curved blade, although now in its modern configuration of advanced steels and synthetic polymers (as opposed to animal bone and horn), continues to maintain its variety of important applications in the field. Even today it is still being used for daily chores such as opening boxes, cutting rope, gardening, construction, working with leather, and for recreational activities like camping, hiking, and fishing.

The modern curved blade, made of contemporary steels and polymers, differs from the curved blade of old only in quality of material. Blade design, length, styles and method of operation have been passed down in the oral tradition from master to student since before recorded history. Those of us fortunate enough to have studied directly under these rare masters, have assumed the responsibility to accurately preserve these ancient teachings in the form of educational media such as DVDs and books (like this one!), training seminars, and of course new curved blade schematics for knife makers based on traditional designs.

The modern curved blade is available in both fixed and folding blade configurations. A fixed blade version has no moving parts, and is far more stable and dependable for almost any application. However, the folding models offer lightweight and compact solutions for modern carry and usage. Additional detail regarding differences between fixed and folding curved blades will be covered in more detail.

Today's curved blade (either fixed or folding) is available in many different shapes and sizes. More important to the overall purpose of this manuscript, though, is the duality in *method of operation* of a curved blade as both a utility knife *and* as a personal safety tool is what sets it apart from other edged tools. As mentioned earlier, the modern curved blade can function as two tools in one—a quality utility knife, and a viable option for personal defense.

CURVED VERSUS STRAIGHT EDGE

What exactly separates a curved blade from a straight blade, aside from obvious geometric differences? Back in the day, one of my early Malaysian teachers taught me a valuable lesson about perspective. There are many ways to look at something and each time you look at it from a different angle (fresh perspective) you learn something new and different about it. According to his philosophy first you observe it with your eyes and then you register it in your brain and this can cause greater under-standing. Thus the more ways you look at something the better you can come to understanding it.

For example, let's work on the idea that you lived your entire exis-tence out in the boonies somewhere and you'd never seen a coffee cup. Upon accidentally finding one, if you looked at it from the bottom you would understand it from that perspective to be a closed cylinder. When you look at it from the top you notice that it is in fact not a closed cylinder but an open one and that it can be used to hold liquids or solids. When you look at it from both sides you notice that it has a thing called a "handle" and that the entire vessel can also be carried by this handle. Thus, again according to the masters, the more changes in your perspective, the greater will your understanding be of that at which you're looking.

The uniqueness and duality of function of the curved blade (more so than a straight blade) can also be viewed from two different perspectives—one as a utility tool and the other as a problem solving tool for personal safety. From these two perspectives we can shed light on at least ten advantages a curved blade has over a straight edge. There are more than these (such as the capability of multiple grips which will be covered later—see "Grips and Mounts"), but for now we will focus on these first ten from two different perspectives.

Utility Tool

Usage of the curved blade as a utility tool goes back centuries, but even today they are found in use by carpet cutters, linoleum tools and installers of other flooring products as well as textiles and other modern functional construction uses.

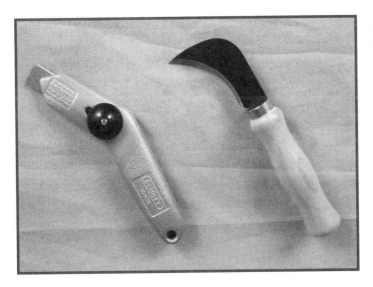

Examples of modern day version of utility tools.

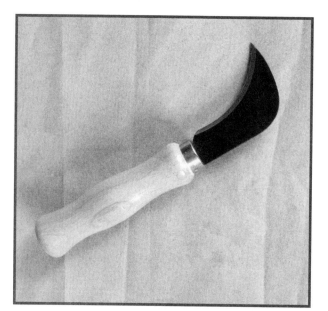

Linoleum Cutter— an example of modern utility usage of the age-old curved blade.

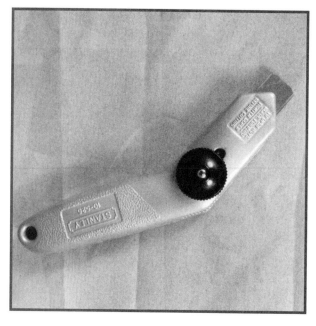

Utility Cutter— yet another example of modern utility usage of the age-old curved blade design.

As was mentioned earlier there are slight advantages of a curved blade over a straight blade as a utility tool. These advantages, with regards to its usage as a utility tool include, but are not limited to the following:

1. It gets a deeper and better bite into the material.

2. The safety ring provides an added level of security so the grip is not compromised.

3. It is easier to manipulate in close quarters and in difficult to reach areas.

4. It can be attached to safety clips or carabineers for safety or storage.

5. Its oversized friction radius (used in addition to the safety ring) helps ensure a positive grip.

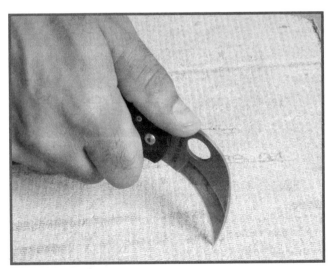

Example of deeper bite into the material as a result of curvature.

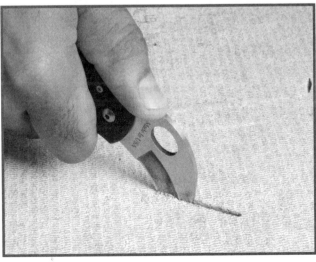

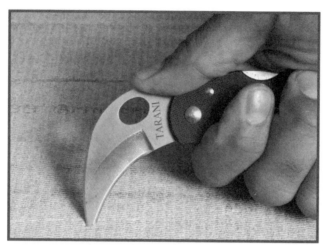

Its oversized friction radius allows for positive thumb placement increasing grip safety.

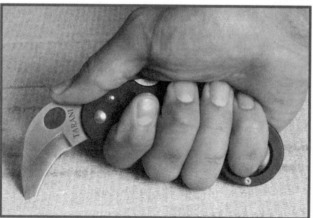

The safety ring provides an added level of security so grip is not compromised.

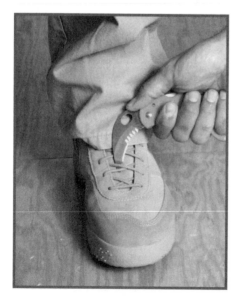

It is easier to manipulate in close quarters and in difficult to reach areas.

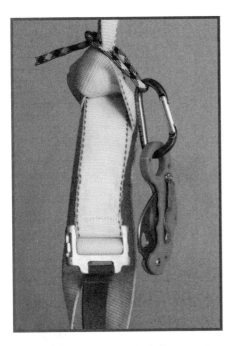

Can be attached to safety clips or carabiner for safety or storage.

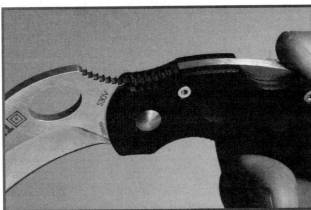

Its oversized friction radius (in addition to the safety ring) ensures positive grip.

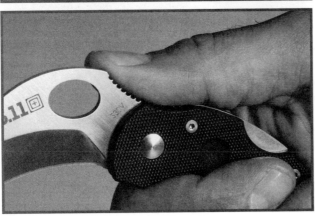

As a utility knife it is superior to other blades in the remarkable safety feature of a finger loop (safety ring) and oversized friction radius so that the blade will not slip in your hand when being used. This significantly reduces the number of self-inflicted injuries as the blade is secured to your finger just like a pair of scissors and will not slip and cut your hand. This especially comes in handy when it's freezing cold outside or if you're underwater, in the rain, in the snow or ice or all of the above!

PERSONAL SAFETY

The utilization of any common edged tool (including a steak knife, butter knife, any kitchen knife or even a plastic knife for that matter), pair of scissors, pen knife or letter opener, can all be used as "implements of opportunity" in personal defense against a violent attacker intent on harming you where your life or limb or that of your loved ones may be at stake.

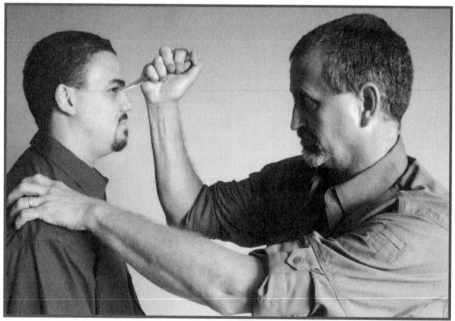

Other tools such as scissors, a pen, or fork can be used both for utility purposes as well as for personal safety and defense.

As was mentioned earlier there are some advantages of a curved blade over a straight blade as a personal safety problem solving tool. These advantages, with regards to its usage as a personal safety tool include, but are not limited to the following:

It cannot be easily seen by your assailant.

It can rapidly change defensive ranges.

It cannot be easily disarmed by the attacker.

It can delivery multiple defensive strikes with a single arm motion.

It can break free or release the deadly weapon arm grip of an attacker in a life-or-death situation should this capability be needed.

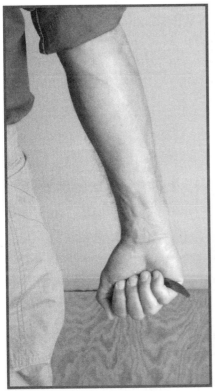
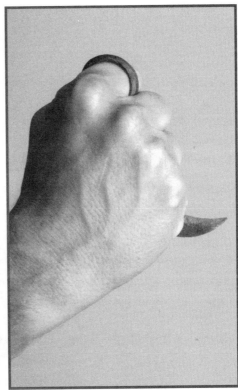

It cannot be easily seen by your opponent.

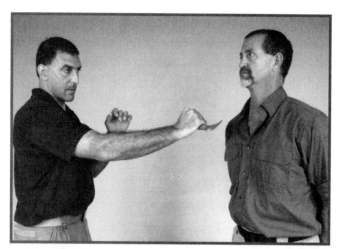

It can rapidly change defensive ranges.

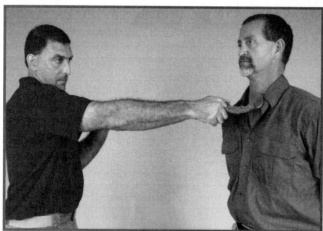

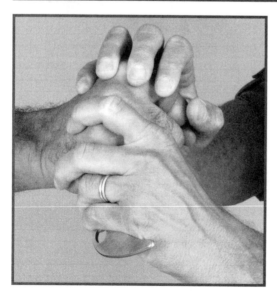

It cannot be easily disarmed by an attacker.

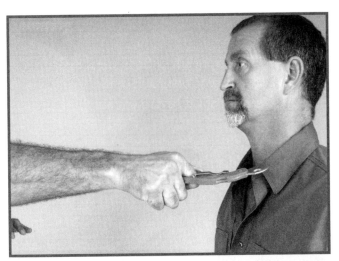

It can deliver multiple defensive strikes with a single arm motion.

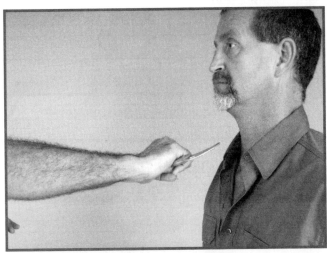

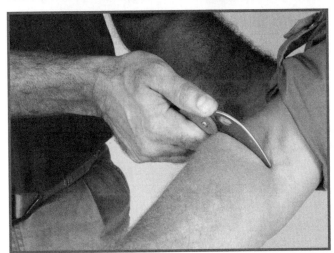

It can break free or release the deadly weapon arm grip of an attacker in a life-or-death situation should this capability be needed.

In the unlikely usage of an edged tool for personal defense, the curved blade is an outstanding option in that it can provide you with both the superiority of a quality blade and an unparalleled functionality which allows additional control of an attacker in a life-or-death altercation providing more options for escape and personal protection than a regular straight edge pocket knife.

Although in modern times most of us do not engage in open battle against heavily armed opponents en masse. We do, however, face the daily threat of single (and sometimes multiple) attackers attempting to relieve us of our daily bread or worse. In such cases, the curved blade can be used as an implement of ensuring personal safety. As a result of its versatile functionality, it is also both a utility tool and a problem-solving tool in everyday life. In fact, more often that not, its sole function is that of a utility tool. Thus, as a result of its multiple applications, ultra-positive gripping features and exceptional operational capabilities, the curved blade is unparalleled in its performance as both a utility tool and "last line" of personal defense.

The curved blade's rich and colorful history, steeped in ancient folklore and unparalleled in functionality, is a testament against the trials of time to its versatility as a utility blade. Coming full circle from its humble origins in the remote villages in West Java and the Southern Philippines, its unique and distinguished design has found its way to the shores of America and into the pockets of knife enthusiasts world wide.

FIXED AND FOLDING

As a direct result of higher demand, the market has responded, through the production of numerous curved blades, with an increase in supply. Today's knife market is flooded with varying shapes, sizes, blade types, and materials in the curved blade arena. There are also varying levels of curved blade quality and functionality both as a utility tool and personal safety tool.

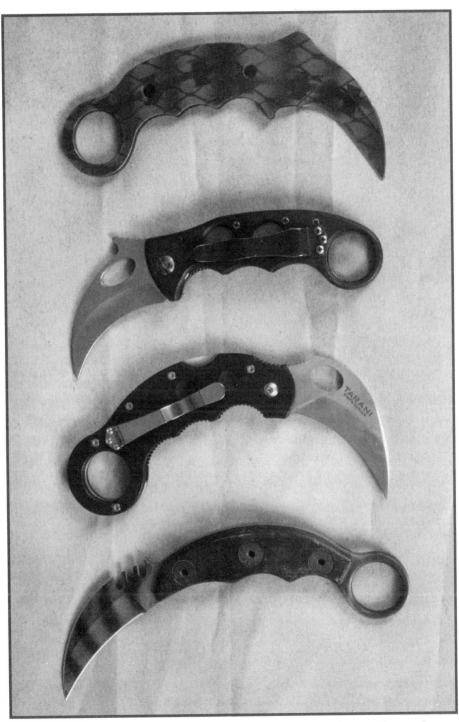

Examples of different curved blades out there on the market today.

What are the differences within this mind-boggling selection of today's curved blades?

The world of curved blades can be divided into two broad categories—fixed and folding. The superior of these two is the fixed version as it is one solid piece of steel and has no moving parts. The immovable handle is affixed to an immovable blade, all hardware is additionally fixed and, naturally, with no moving parts fewer things can go wrong.

It is often said that everything has a price tag and the price tag for a fixed curved blade is that although superior in craftsmanship, functionality and material, it can sometimes be inconvenient to carry. Fixed curved blades tend to be larger and more difficult to carry on your person when, for example, at a business meeting or driving in your car for long periods of time, or when running or walking the dogs. Most of the fixed models are designed for immediate access and the price for that feature is that it may not be as convenient to carry as a folding model.

In my opinion, Strider Knives are the highest quality fixed curved blade on the market as of this writing. Given the highest grade and heat-treat of steel available (CPM S30V) and the multiple position carry systems available to sheath the blade, it's a pretty easy choice.

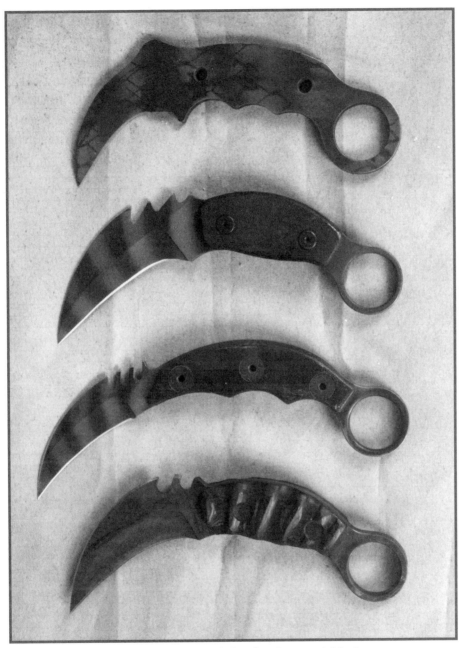

Example of some of the fixed curved blades
offered by Strider Knives Inc.

Folders are lightweight (lighter than fixed), easier to carry, can be carried in more places (given limited available real-estate on the human body), are easy to manipulate and can be just as immediately effective as the fixed blade once they are deployed. Generally the handles are of lightweight scales such as G10, FRN or some other polymer and are conducive to convenient carry and storage since they require no carry system. A great variety of these are now available via 5.11 Tactical (which I consider to be of superior quality), SpyderCo, Emerson and a variety of other production knife makers. For a more comprehensive listing click on www.karambit.com.

While being lighter in weight and convenient to carry are the upside of folding curved blades, the downside is that they have moving parts as a function of their design and require additional deployment steps. Nonetheless, convenience and lightweight carry remain important options.

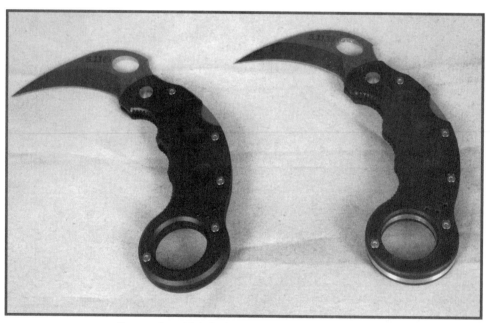

Example of high-quality folding curved blades
offered by 5.11 tactical.

Another difference between fixed and folding curved blades is the curvature of the blade itself. Since fixed blades are sheathed and the blade is completely contained within the carry system, a fixed curved blade may safely hold a double edge. On the other side of the fence, since in the closed (unlocked) position, more than half of a folding curved blade is exposed, it cannot be double edged.

Additionally, there is a traditional "fork" shape of the blade at the base of the curve located just above the handle of the fixed curved blade which is completely covered by the carry system. Again, due to the functionality of the folding curved blade design it is not possible for this feature to be included.

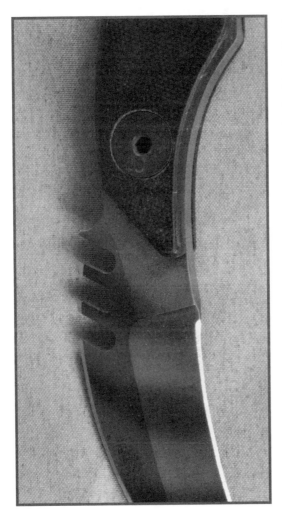

Fixed blades are sheathed and the blade is completely contained within the carry system, a fixed curved blade may safely hold a double edge.

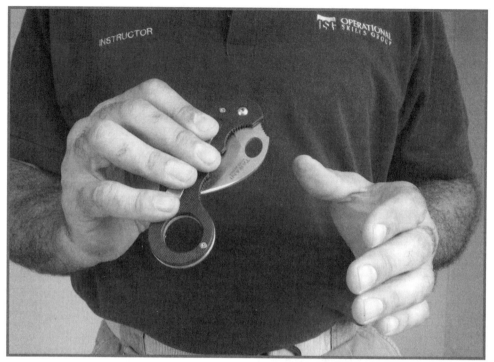

Since more than half of the blade is exposed on folding curved blades they cannot be double edged.

When deciding whether to go with a fixed model or a folding model it's important to understand and be aware of the differences between the two and that there are advantages and disadvantages to each. Due to popular demand (numerous questions regarding usage of the folding curved blade by my students around the world) the scope of study for the remainder of this manuscript will be focused primarily on the folding curved blade.

SELECTION

When selecting a curved blade the first consideration should be form fitting function. That is, what is the intended use for your curved blade? Will it be used to open boxes, cut linoleum or carpet, for construction or building purposes, to augment your personal safety options, impressing your neighbors, personal collection only? All of the above? None of the above? These are all important factors when it comes time to selecting the curved blade of your choice.

Your hand size is also a consideration with regards to the length of the handle and the diameter of the safety ring. More info on the safety ring will be covered later, but for now some important questions would include: Do you have large or small hands? Will you be wearing gloves? Are your fingers thick or thin, long or short? Could the curved blade be used in inclement weather? Underwater? In adverse conditions? In a dry and arid desert environment? Would you be wearing gloves? These questions again are extremely subjective and can only be answered by the buyer.

Some good questions regarding selection have come up over the years—such as the angle of the blade and the length and the shape and why a fixed blade has less of a curve than a folding blade and the concept of single edged and double edged and false edge, handle length and the diameter of the ring. Let's take a closer look at each of these individually to gain a better perspective.

PARTS

The modern curved blade consists of nine characteristic parts each uniquely contributing to overall functionality and quality of blade design.

Since there are two distinct configurations of any curved blade—fixed and folding, the following illustrations provide a breakdown of each.

These nine characteristic parts of the traditional fixed curved blade include:

1. Inside Edge

2. Outside Edge (some versions and styles do not have an outside edge)

3. Point

4. Barb (some versions have a barb and some do not)

5. Blade Shaft

6. Handle

7. Front Brake

8. Rear Brake

9. Safety ring

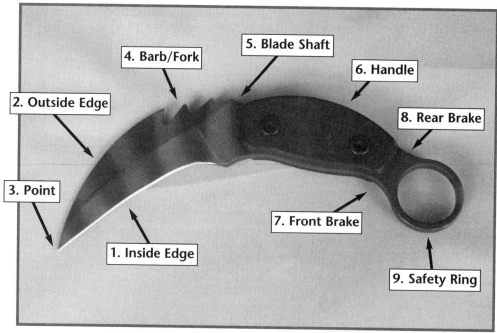

1. Inside Edge, 2. Outside Edge (some versions and styles do not have an outside edge), 3. Point, 4. Barb (again, some have a barb and some do not or is purposely rounded depending on blade type), 5. Blade Shaft, 6. Handle, 7. Front Brake, 8. Rear Brake, and 9. Safety ring.

There are also nine characteristic parts of the modern folding curved blade which include:

1. Inside Edge

2. False Edge

3. Point

4. Friction Radius

5. Blade Shaft

6. Handle

7. Front Brake

8. Rear Brake

9. Safety ring

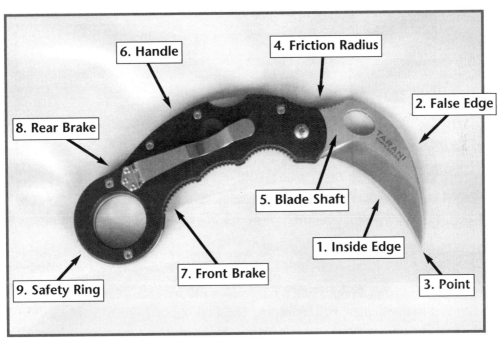

1. Inside Edge, 2. False Edge 3. Point, 4. Friction Radius,
5. Blade Shaft, 6. Handle, 7. Front Brake, 8. Rear Brake,
and lastly the 9. Safety ring.

Blade Angle

The blade of either a fixed or folding curved blade knife can be of any length or curvature. Sometimes mistakenly called an "angle," the curvature of a blade varies depending on both the manufacturer and the blade's intended functionality.

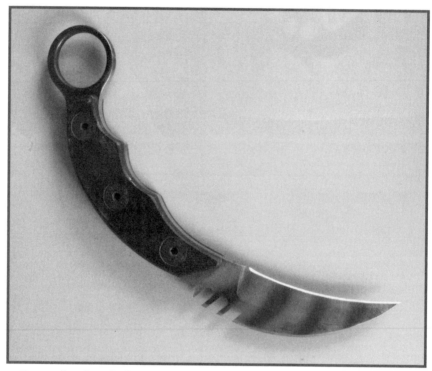

Example of a shallow curve—traditional in fixed blade designs.

Generally speaking a fixed blade will have less curvature (more of a shallow angle) than a folding blade because it must be stored and retrieved from a carry system by way of sheath fully covering all parts of the blade. Partly by design and partly by function, too much of a curvature and deploying the straight blade from its carry system would not be practical. Too straight of a curve also diminishes the functionality of the curve and compromises the integrity of the advantages of a curved blade both for utilitarian and personal safety application.

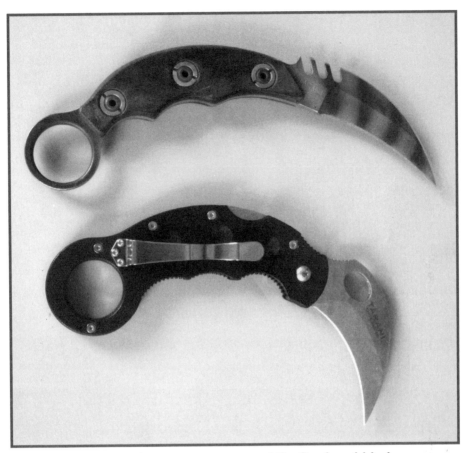

Difference between curvature of the fixed and blade.

Generally speaking, a quality folding curved blade allows for more of a curve as it does not require a carry system (sheath). In the industry, with regards to the folding model, due to production costs, it's generally easier (and less costly) to manufacture a "straight" curved folding blade than it is a true curved folding blade as there is considerable engineering that goes into a true quality deeply curved folding blade design. As with most quality folding curved blades, the deeper the curve, the more time and money that went into the design and manufacture, and if high-end steels and handle materials (such as CPM S30V or 154CM with G10 scales) the higher the quality.

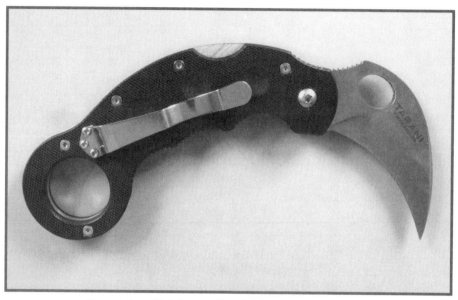

Example of high-quality folding curved blade.

Single vs. Double Edged

The difference between single edged and double edged models is that a double edge requires complete coverage of the blade whereas the single edge version does not. Although not all fixed curved blades are double edge, all fixed curved blades have the capacity to hold a double edge given that the blade is completely covered by the sheath.

Folding curved blades do not have that option as the majority of the blade is exposed due to the knife's basic functionality. Although it is possible to sharpen the very tip of the blade that may be covered in between the handle, it is not advised in the event that the blade may open inadvertently in your pocket or other carry position.

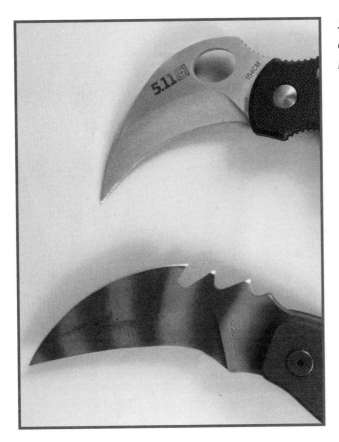

Single edged versus double edged folding curved blade.

Single versus double edged is yet another consideration in selection and purchase of a curved blade as the laws regarding knives in certain states do not permit citizens to own double edged blades.

Handle Length

Along with the various selections of curved blades available comes a variety of handle lengths as well. Simply stated, the length of the handle should closely match the width of the palm of your hand. The proximity of the base of the blade to the edge of the safety ring should be sufficient enough to fit the measurement of your hand in a closed fist position.

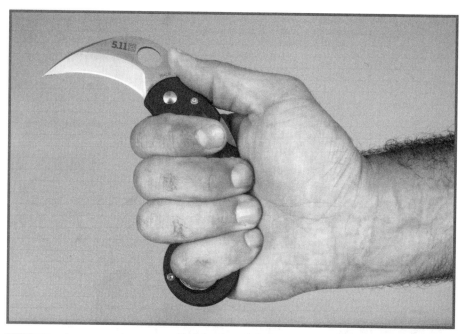

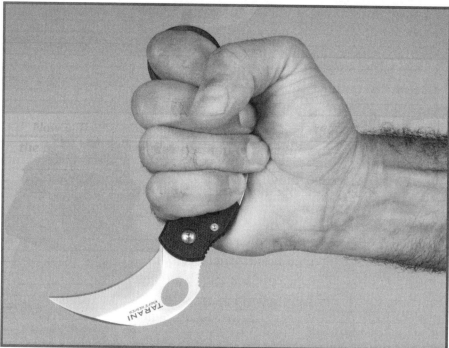

The length of your hand should fit comfortably in both blade up and blade down configurations with adequate space between the base of the curved blade and the edge of the safety ring.

Safety Ring

One of the most unique and characteristic features of the curved blade is the safety ring. The safety ring provides an added measure of security when utilizing the blade both as a utility tool and as a personal safety tool. This unique feature of the curved blade prevents slippage of the knife blade in the hand when either pushing or pulling the handle in any direction. The added security of the safety ring also allows for a more positive grip and considerable application of blade edge and tip force in a safe and controlled manner.

The safety ring traditionally measures 1" in diameter. Various knife companies manufacture different safety ring diameters based on customer demand. Ring size is completely subjective and is a matter of personal comfort. However, if the ring is too tight or it is the case that you know you will only be using this knife when wearing gloves, then it's

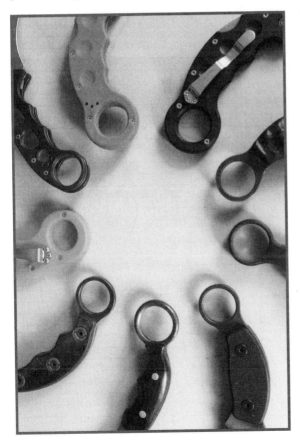

necessary to shop around for a larger ring. If the opposite is true and your finger swims around in the ring then it may be the case that a smaller safety ring diameter is needed. Usage of the safety ring while properly mounting and gripping the blade will be covered in more detail later on, but strictly for purposes of curved blade selection and personal fit, the ring should be easily mounted and dismounted.

Examples of various curved blade Safety Rings.

CARRY

Fixed curved blades are always carried with a sheath which safely covers both the edge and the tip fully protecting the carry position. The carry system of any fixed curved blade can be worn on the outside (not concealed) high and low rise, behind the waistband, around the neck and strapped on to external gear such as load bearing vests and the like. Fixed curved blades can also be concealed by means such as neck carry or under garments. Be sure to confirm this method of carry is in compliance with state and local laws.

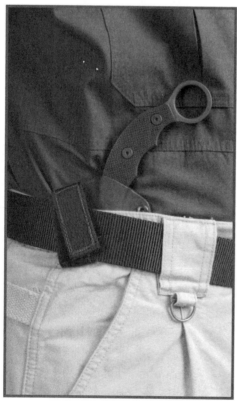

*Fixed curved blade
tip-down carry.*

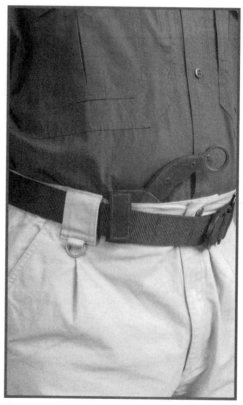

*Fixed curved blade
same-side front carry.*

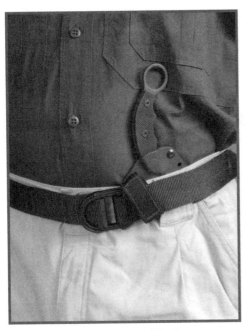

*Fixed curved blade
cross-body front carry.*

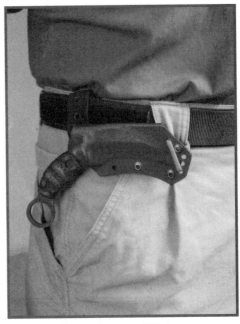

*Fixed curved blade
tip-up carry.*

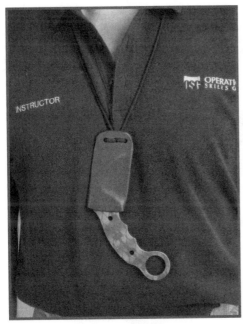

*Fixed curved blade
neck carry.*

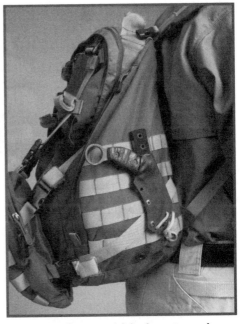

*Fixed curved blade external
carry, load bearing vest.*

Although some folders come with a sheath, the vast majority are available with a carry clip. In most cases this clip is ambidextrous and can be worn on either side of the body or pocket carry.

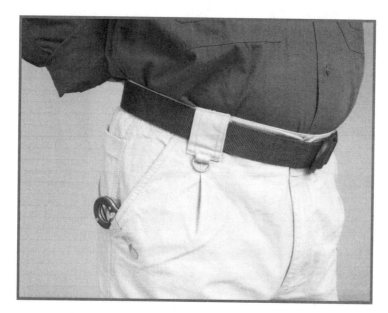

Folding curved blade right pocket carry.

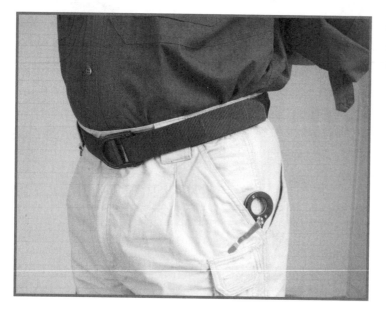

Folding curved blade left pocket carry.

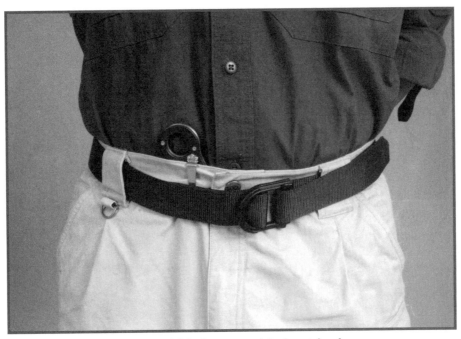

Folding curved blade same-side front body carry.

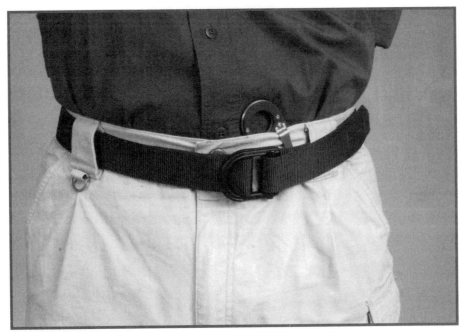

Folding curved blade cross-body front carry.

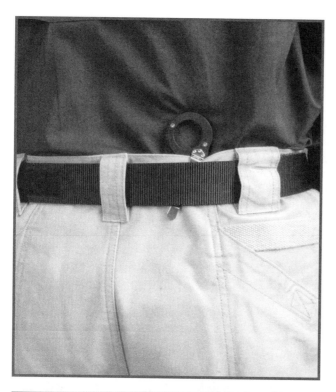

Folding curved blade same-side rear body carry.

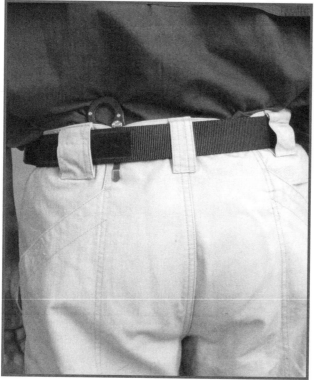

Folding curved blade cross-body rear carry.

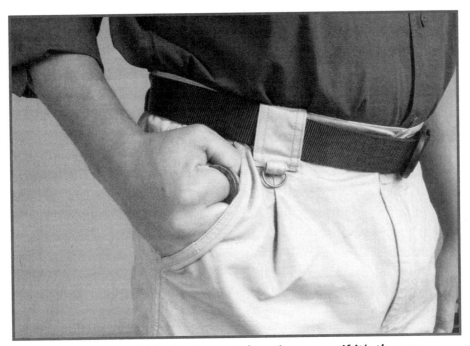

Folding curved blade alternate location carry. If it's the case that you have perceived an imminent threat the blade can also be unsheathed or locked into the open position and in your hand inside your pocket or suit coat or purse.

The key to curved blade carry—whether fixed or folding is *accessibility to the hands*. This is similar to handgun holsters; the position of the holster is placed in immediate proximity to the hands. In the event the curved blade (and its usage as personal defense tool) may be needed, this close proximity allows for expedient acquisition of grip and deployment from the carry position as well as the ability to assume a defensive posture in a relatively short period of time.

Grip and deployment of the curved blade for purposes of personal safety will be covered in more detail later in our study.

LOCK AND UNLOCK

Locking and unlocking the curved blade is another way of referring to "opening" and "closing" the knife. A fixed blade is in a constant locked, open position and there is nothing to do but remove it from its sheath and return it to its sheath.

The folding curved blade is a different matter and in fact locking and unlocking require specific handling. It is important to note that a folding curved blade that is partially open (not in the locked position) can be tremendously hazardous to the safety of fingers. It is strongly recommended that a curved blade be either fully locked (open) or safely unlocked (closed).

Locking

There are as many different locking mechanisms available as there are different curved blade models. The two most common locking mechanisms of the folding curved blade are the liner lock and the back lock.

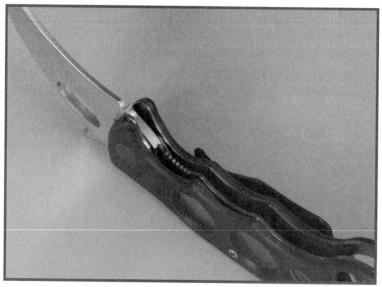

Folding curved blade example of a liner lock.

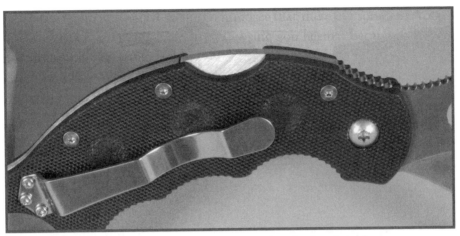

Folding curved blade example of a back lock.

The mechanics of locking and unlocking the curved folding blade are simple. The blade moves away from the handle (or the handle moves away from the blade) guided by the pivot point located at the base of the blade and the top part of the handle, from an unlocked and closed position (meaning the folding knife as it is at rest "folded") toward a locked and open position.

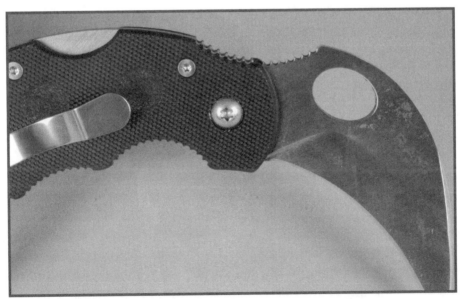

Close-up of a pivot screw which guides the blade
between the locked and unlocked positions.

The safety issues regarding operation of a folding curved blade are, of course, safeguarding against unintentional contact with the edge and tip of the curved blade. With the blade in the folded (unlocked) position there is little or no risk of injury. However, the instant the blade begins to move from its closed position out to the open and finally in the locked position, is the time when risk of personal injury is greatest.

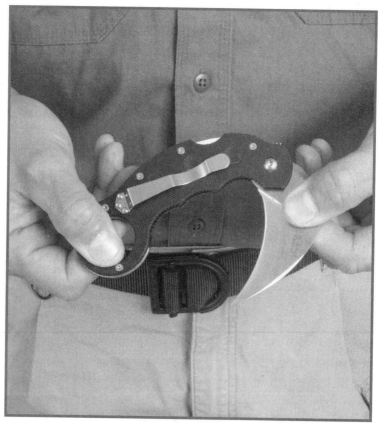

Potential for personal injury begins as soon as the blade and tip are exposed.

The steps to safely locking the blade in the open position are to utilize the opening mechanism of the blade in such a manner as to bring the blade out fully away from the handle until you can make both visual and tactile confirmation that the locking mechanism is engaged.

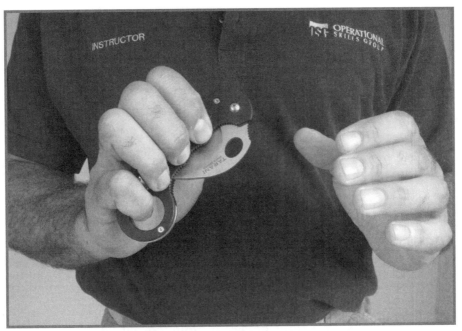

*Begin with the blade in one hand, in the closed position
with both hands in front of your body.*

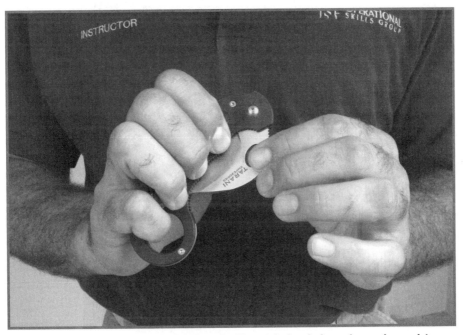

*Grasp the curved blade folding knife with both hands and reaching
for the opening mechanism with your support (non-dominant) hand.*

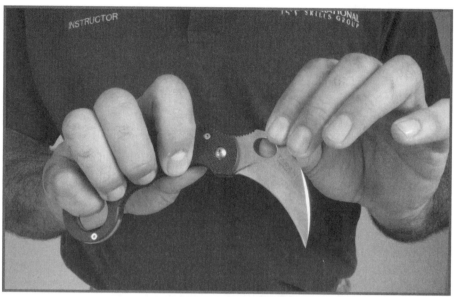

Utilize the opening mechanism (in this case an oval machined out of the blade) to begin moving the blade from its closed (unlocked) position.

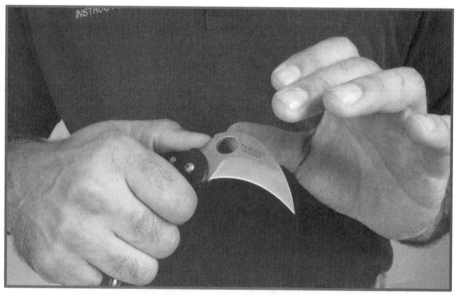

Extend the blade in such a manner as to bring the blade fully away from the handle out until you can make both visual and tactile confirmation that the locking mechanism is engaged.

Unlocking

Safety being paramount, the unlocking of any curved blade can be especially dangerous to the fingers. Similar to the function of a cigar cutter, the closing of a curved blade directly upon the fingers can have devastating consequences. It is critical that nothing remain in between the path of the blade and the handle opening to receive the blade during the unlocking and "closing" of the blade movement.

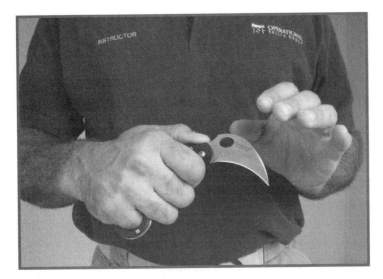

Begin with the blade in one hand and in the opened position with both hands in front of your body.

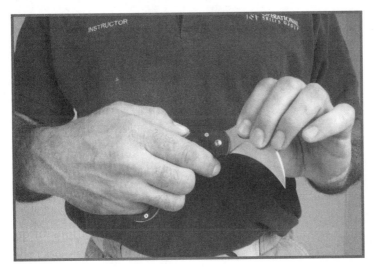

Grasp the curved blade folding knife with both hands in the open or locked position.

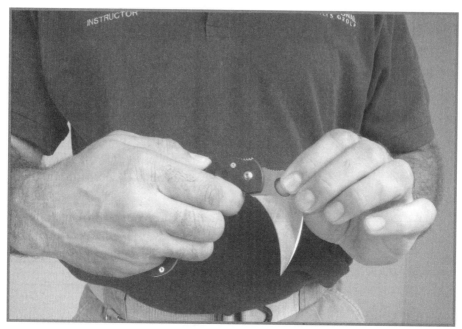

Disengage the locking mechanism.

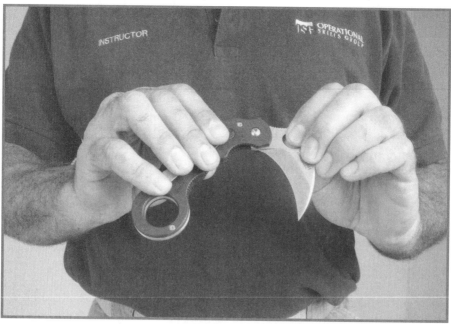

Turn the edge and tip away from your body.

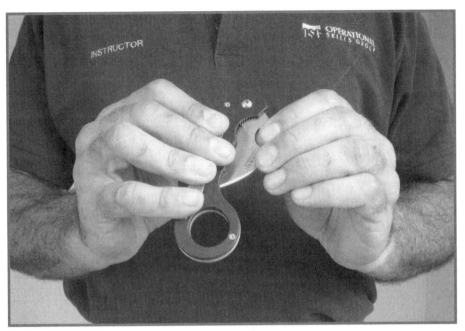

Remove any digits from the path of the closing blade.

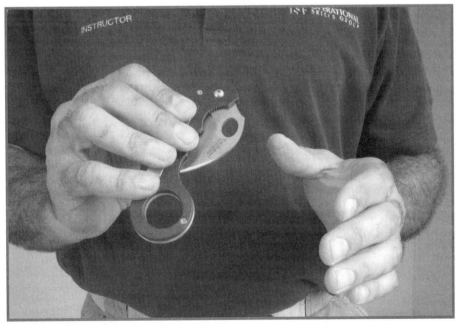

Safely close the blade into the handle with visual confirmation.

The key to safely utilizing any folding curved blade for both utility and personal safety purposes is the ability to safely and securely open and close the blade. In the event of a personal safety situation, the blade must not only be easily accessible, safely locked and unlocked (opened and closed) but also rapidly deployed which will be covered later.

GRIPS AND MOUNTS

Since the curved blade is such a unique and specific design, the defining characteristics (curved blade, safety ring, and oversized friction radius) warrant specific handling. Before the blade can be used for either utility or personal safety purposes, a sound working knowledge of how to mount (place the knife in position on your hand) and grip (hold on to) the knife is required.

Additionally, given the uniqueness of the curvature of the blade and (as is the case of any quality curved blade) curvature of the handle, specific grip and mounting techniques are better suited than others for blade handling.

It's a curved blade and most likely a curved handle which is very different than the usual straight handle and straight blade, so how do you hold on to the thing?

The mantra here with regards to grips, mounts and overall blade usage is "form fits function." There are a number of ways in which to grip the curved blade, however, before a grip can be acquired it is necessary to "mount" the knife—which is a training term meaning "to place it into your grip." The two (grips and mounts) are mutually dependant as one must first decide which grip will be utilized and the mount will be determined by the grip.

Grips

As mentioned earlier there are about a dozen differences between the usage of curved blades and straight blades applied both as a utility tool and as a problem solving tool in the event of a personal defense situation. Another of the major differences between the two blade types is the manner in which the knife may be gripped.

If you are the proud owner of a straight blade (fixed or folding) there are only two specific grips that are permitted by the geometric shape of the blade (a straight edge with a straight handle) and those are: blade forward (up) or blade reversed (down).

Of course for you knife aficionados out there, there may be some variations on these two grips such as fingers or thumbs off to the side of the handle or the blade, but the tip of the straight blade, based on the straight handle, can only be in one of two directions—tip up or tip down.

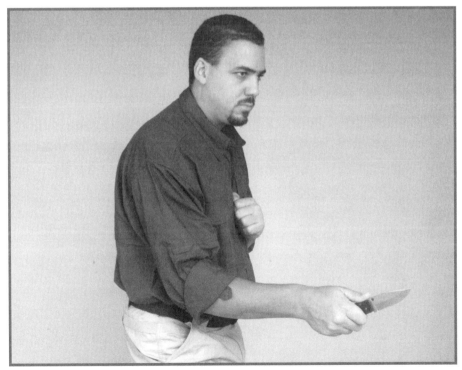

Straight edge grip—blade up (or forward) configuration.

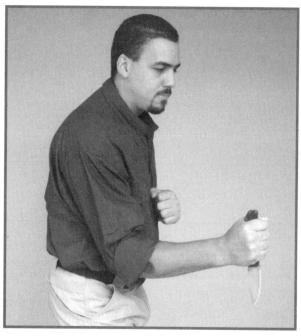

*Straight edge grip—
tip down configura-
tion with edge
facing forward.*

Yes, there are minor variations of these two such as (if we're discussing a *single* edged straight blade) the blade edge facing forward or blade edge facing back, or maybe the thumb is resting on the knife or the thumb is resting on your other fingers, etc. The bottom line is that the geometry of a straight edge blade again allows for only two general grips—blade up or blade down.

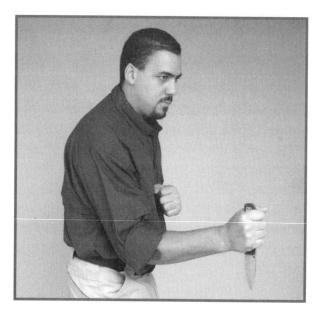

*Straight edge grip—
tip down configura-
tion with edge
facing backward
and thumb on the
side of the handle.*

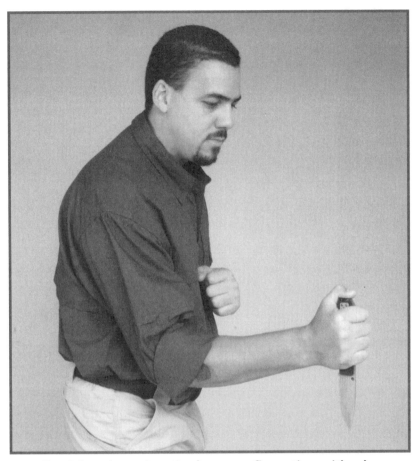

*Straight edge grip—tip down configuration with edge
facing backward and thumb on top of the handle.*

If you are the proud owner of a curved blade (fixed or folding) there are *three* specific grips that are permitted by the geometric shape of the blade (a curved edge with a curved handle) as well as the unique characteristics of the curved folding knife (e.g. safety ring and oversized friction radius) and those are: blade forward (up), blade reversed (down) and blade extended (out).

The three (3) grip configurations unique to the curved blade:

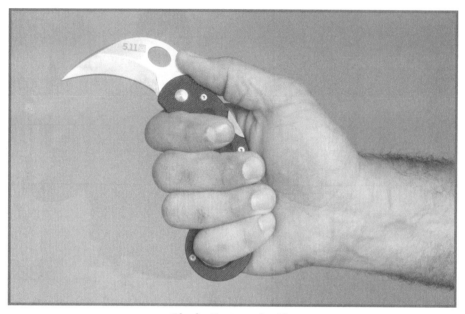

Blade Forward—Up

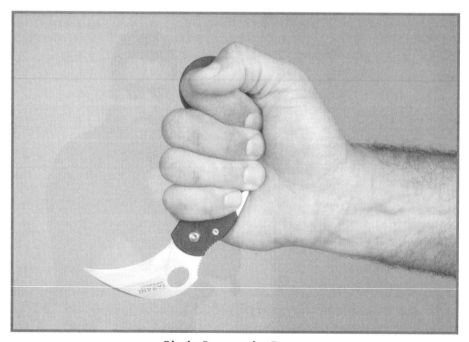

Blade Reversed—Down

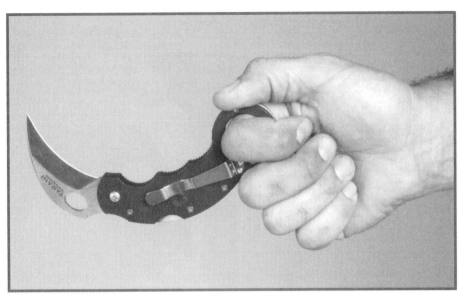

Blade Extended—Out

Similar to the straight edge grip the thumb may either be placed on the knife or on the hand, whichever is more comfortable.

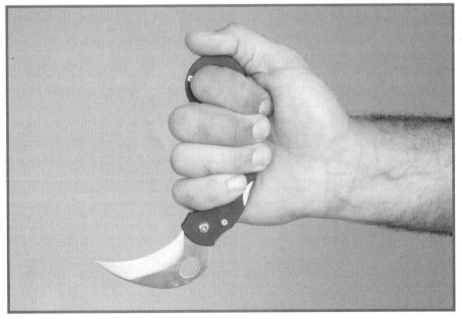

Thumb rest on Safety Ring—blade in retracted position.

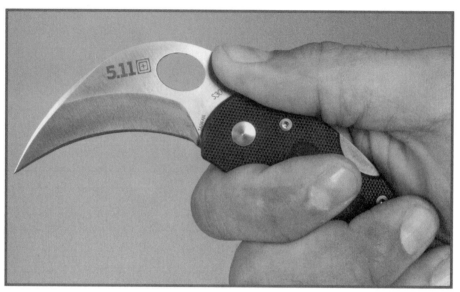

Thumb rest on friction radius—blade forward (tip up).

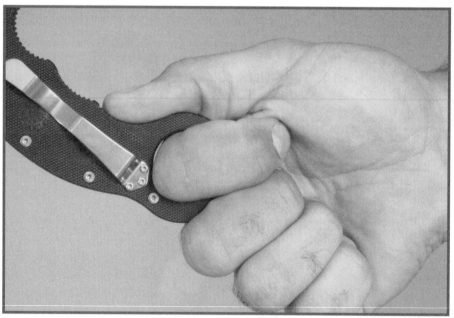

Thumb rest on front break—blade in extended position.

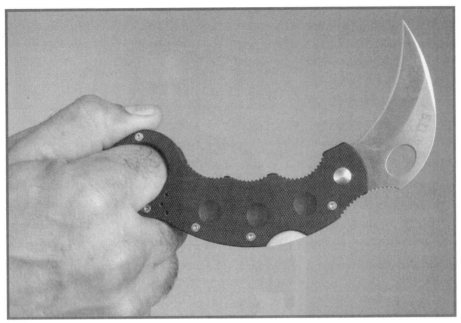

Thumb rest on safety ring—blade in extended position.

Mounts

The carry location, curved blade type (fixed or folding), access to the knife, acquisition of optimal grip and the grip, all determine the mount. The mount is just another term referring to the manner in which the blade is held in the hand. There are two types of mounts—the Grip Mount and the Safety Mount.

Grip Mounts

Again, for purposes of both utility and self-defense, once the curved blade has been fixed into a grip of your choice, it can be mounted for usage in any one of three possible configurations. These are gripping the blade in the vertical palm position, gripping the blade in the palm down position and gripping the blade in the palm up position. As will be covered in greater detail later, all three of these grip mounts can provide the user optimal response based on position and circumstance.

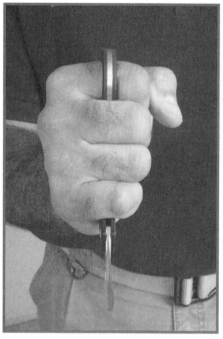

Grip mounted in the palm vertical configuration.

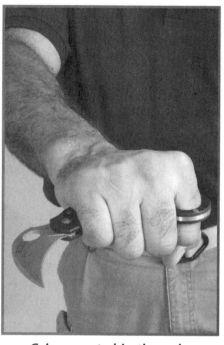

Grip mounted in the palm down configuration.

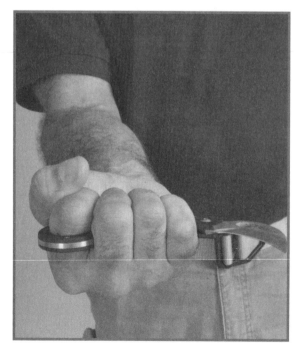

Grip mounted in the palm up configuration.

Safety Mounts

Prior to determining the position of the palm when gripping the curved blade (Grip Mounts), it is first necessary to mount the curved blade into the hand utilizing the safety ring in such a manner as to affix the blade to the hand as safely as possible to prevent loss of the blade during application. This safely securing or mounting the blade to your hand is often referred to as the Safety Mount.

As covered previously, unlike all other hand-held blades, the curved blade with its unique safety ring allows for three mounted positions—tip up or tip down retracted and also extended. But how do you actually mount the blade in such a manner as to safely manipulate it with your hand?

Starting with the safest and most powerful grip—tip up (or forward), let's take a closer look at the procedure for safely mounting a curved blade resulting in the tip up configuration.

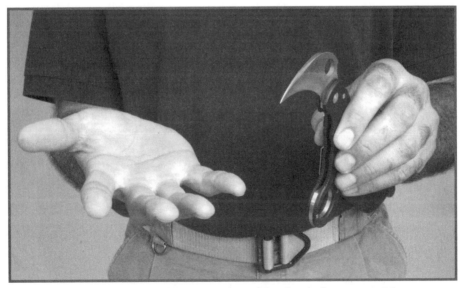

Begin with your dominant hand in the palm up position and holding the curved blade (either fixed or locked open folding) in your other hand.

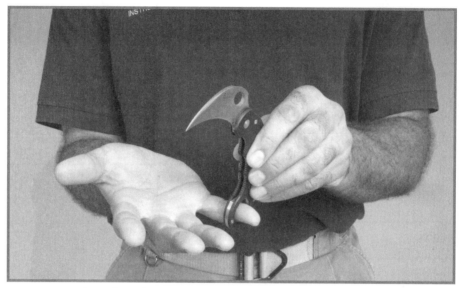

Keeping the edge and tip facing forward and away from your body, place your little finger into the Safety Ring.

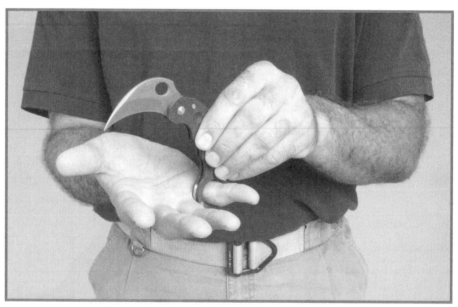

Continue to move the baby finger forward until a firm placement of the safety ring is achieved by moving the ring up high and pressing into the web of skin between the ring finger and little finger. Remember to keep the edge and tip pointing away from any of your body parts.

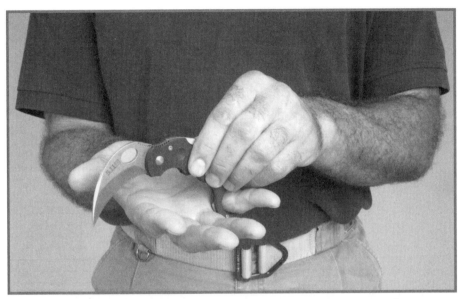

*Angle the blade down and away from your center so that
while pivoting on the safety ring the top of the handle
rotates toward your index finger.*

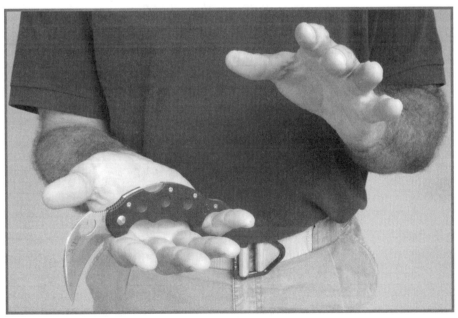

*Release the blade from your support hand and let gravity
take the weight of the steel and allow it to rest naturally
in the palm of your open hand.*

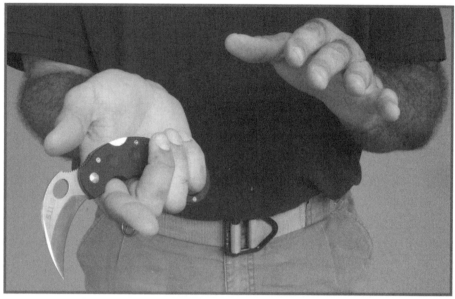

After it settles into the natural shape of your personal grip, beginning with your little finger, start to form a seal around the handle with your four fingers. Start at the safety ring and moving forward to the blade.

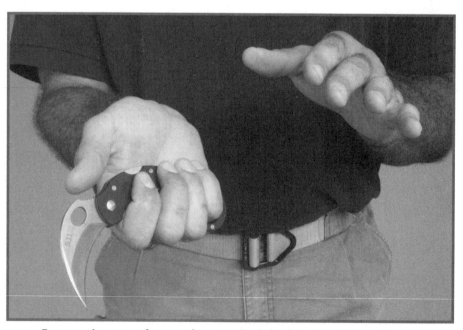

For maximum safety and control of the blade, all four fingers should be firmly in place grasping the handle.

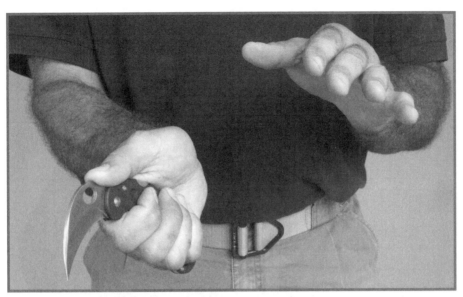

After the fingers are locked into a comfortable position then place your strong-side thumb onto the friction radius.

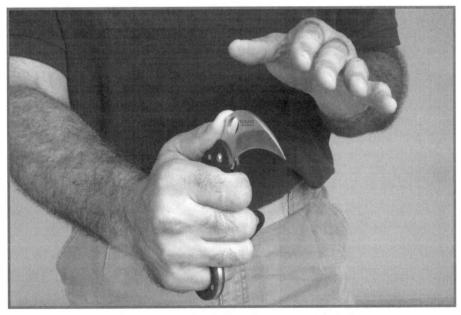

In order to complete the full Safety Mount it is important to keep your support hand safely behind and away from the edge and tip of the curved blade. From this Safety Mount you may then move to any of the three grip mounts you want—palm vertical, palm down or palm up.

Moving to the next Safety Mount—blade tip facing downward, let's take a closer look at the steps required to achieve this mount.

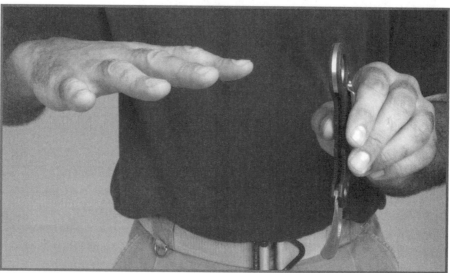

Begin with your dominant hand in the palm down position and holding the curved blade (either fixed or locked open folding) in your other hand.

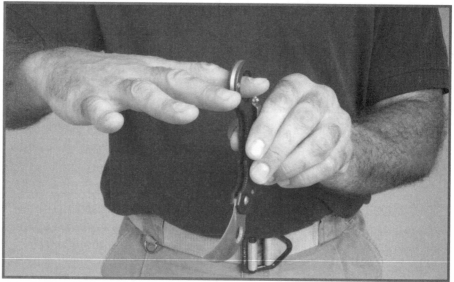

Keeping the edge and tip facing forward and away from your body, place your index finger into the Safety Ring.

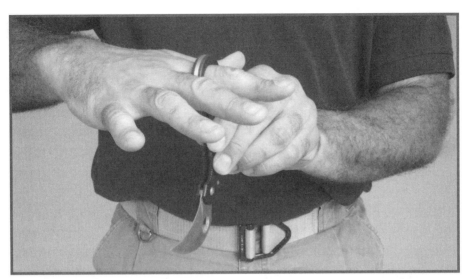

Continue to move your index finger forward until a firm placement of the safety ring is achieved by moving the ring up high and pressing into the web of skin between the index and middle fingers. Remember to keep the edge and tip pointing away from any of your own body parts.

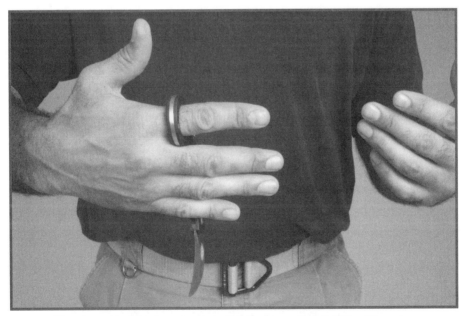

Allowing the blade to swing freely from the Safety Ring, turn your palm inward toward your body and allow the blade handle to align with and rest lightly against your remaining fingers.

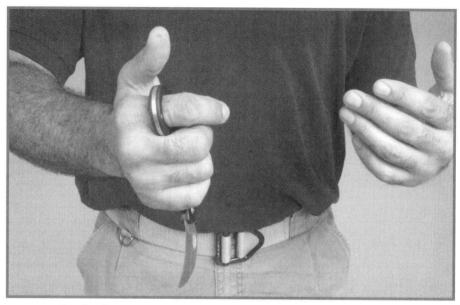

*Beginning again with the little finger, form a tight seal
around the handle with all fingers.*

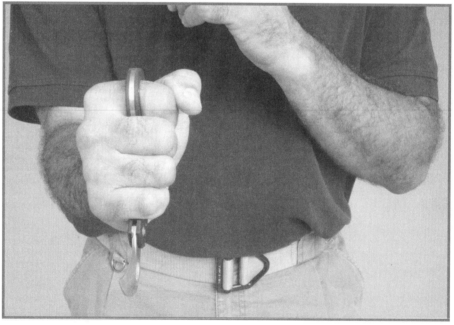

*Finish the seal with your thumb (which can either rest on
the Safety Ring or on the side of your own hand, as pictured),
thus completing the Safety Mount.*

Spinning

Sure looks good in the movies and for stage demonstrations but in real life it's not such a good idea—especially in the event that you may need to really use the curved blade for personal safety.

Similar to a straight edge knife, the action of flipping it back and forth in your hand removes the blade from any useful position of application. Again, this may deeply impress your friends and family at Thanksgiving dinner, but while you're in the process of flipping back and forth the fight is on, the attacker is taking advantage of your down time. Unfortunately that's what's spinning—the clock.

Once you're in a particular position (Grip Mount)—stay in that position and fight from that position until you can reach a point that you are able—and have made the conscious decision to change your grip.

Should it be the case that you have a lull in the action and you can afford a bit of down time, then here's how you would go about changing blade position by flipping the curved blade in your hand—otherwise known as "spinning."

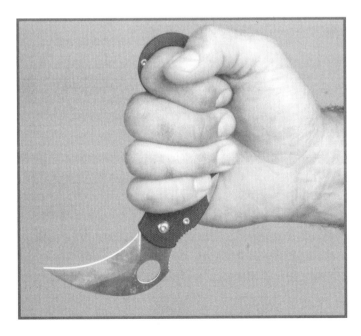

Start from the retracted position with blade pointing down.

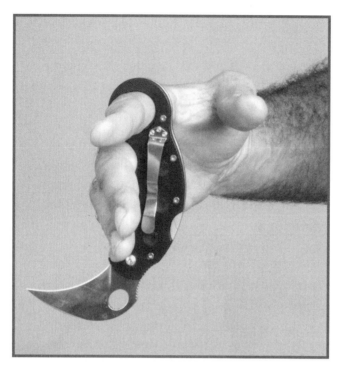

Reversing the steps of a Safety Mount, release your fingers and let the curved blade hang lightly against your fingers supported only by the Safety Ring.

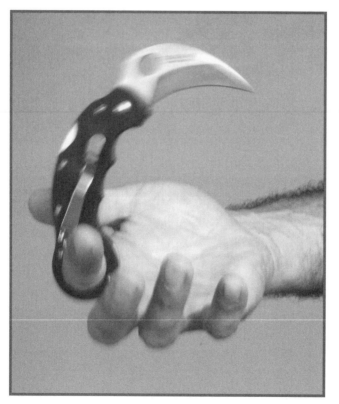

Pushing your hand away from you in a fashion similar to shooing a fly, allow the blade to roll OVER your index finger guided by the Safety Ring.

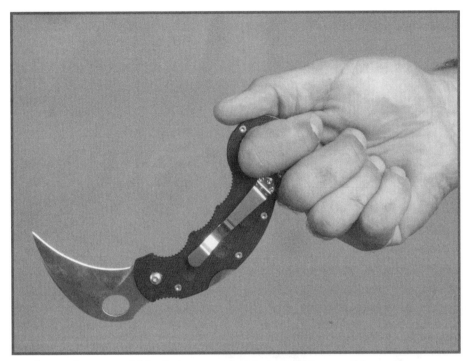

Once the curved blade is extended (you will know this as the rear break should now be pressing the weight of the curved blade against your middle finger), you may place your thumb either on the Safety Ring (as illustrated) or alongside the ring against your own hand.

In case you may be wondering, as this is a frequently asked question, it is only possible to spin the curved blade from the Blade Down configuration and not the Blade Up configuration.

READY POSITIONS

Once the blade is safely mounted in your position of choice, you may then move your hand with the mounted blade to any number of Ready Positions from which you may apply the curved blade. For purposes of both utility and personal safety application there are a total of five Ready Positions.

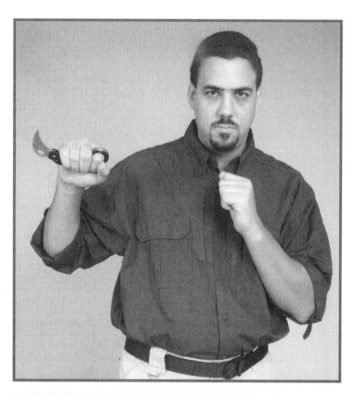

*High Open
Position*

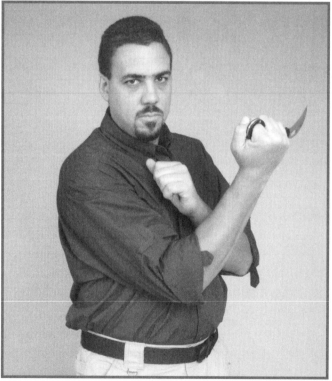

*High Closed
Position*

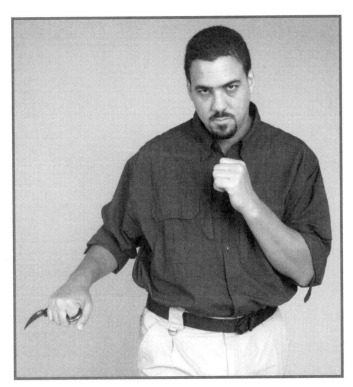

*Low Open
Position*

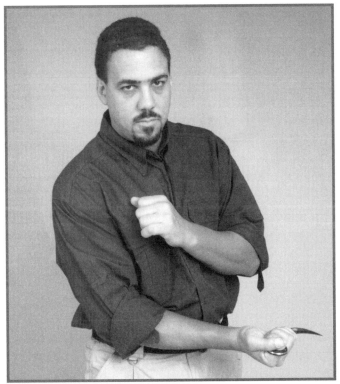

*Low Closed
Position*

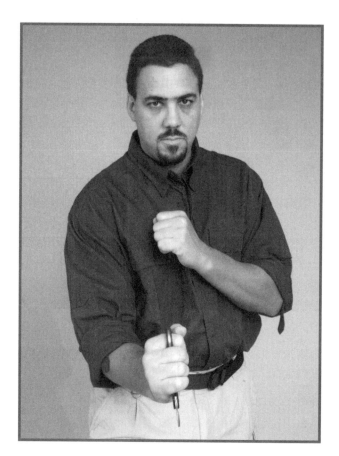

*Low Guard
Position*

DEPLOYMENT

Literally the word "deployment," when utilized for description of curved blade use (or any knife for that matter), simply refers to "removing the tool from its carry position," unlocking or unsheathing, mounting, gripping and moving to a position in which to utilize the blade whether it be as a utility tool or for personal defense and safety.

Rapid Deployment

In the event of a personal safety situation, the faster you are able to access your curved blade the better. Another fancy term for quickly accessing and removing your curved blade from its carry position is "rapid deployment." Depending upon whether it is a fixed or folding curved blade there are varying methods of rapid deployment. Let's first take a look at the fixed curved blade.

Superior to the folding curved blade (by virtue of no moving parts), there is really little or nothing to do other than to remove it from its carry position which will always be from a sheath or "carry system."

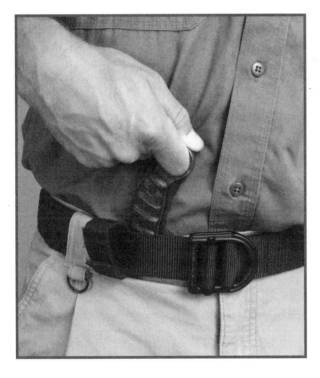

Forefinger Safety Ring grasp—example of fixed blade deployment.

There's no secret to fixed curved blade rapid deployment other than immediate access to carry position and deploy that edge as smoothly as possible.

The real trick comes when deploying a folding curved blade since it has moving parts and although no carry system, it still needs to be accessed by the hands, removed from its carry position and then moved from the unlocked (closed) position to the locked (open) position in a safe and timely manner. Here's where we need to take a closer look at rapid deployment of the folding curved blade.

There are two methods of deploying the folding curved blade. One is with the tip upward, or "standard grip" and the other with the tip facing downward otherwise known as "reverse grip." The more difficult of these methods is the blade tip facing upward as it is the most powerful mount and grip. The price tag is that it takes maybe an additional ? or ? second or so to execute.

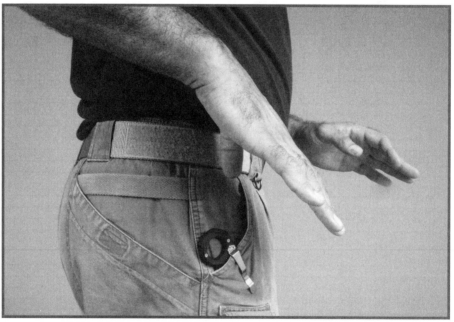

Starting from dominant hand side (strong side) in the example right pocket carry, begin with your hand above the pocket line.

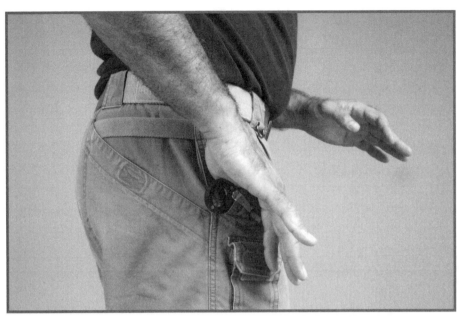

Inserting your thumb into the pocket, press aggressively to gain a deep seated initial grip by pressing hard enough to catch the web of skin between your thumb and forefinger.

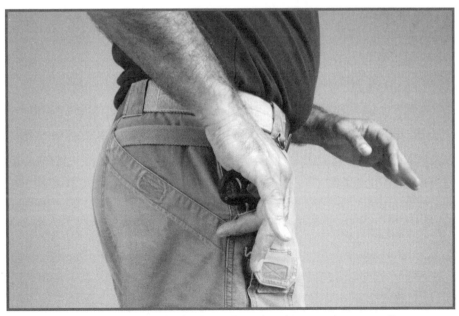

Once your thumb is locked in place begin to wrap your fingers around the handle to acquire a positive grip.

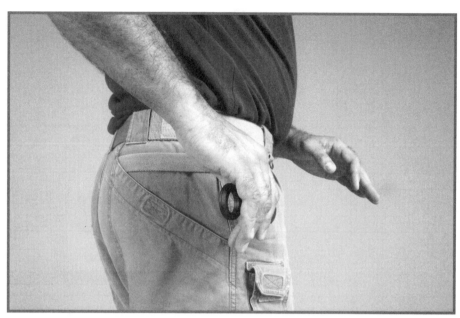

Upon acquisition of positive grip on the folding curved blade handle you may now begin to remove the knife from its carry position.

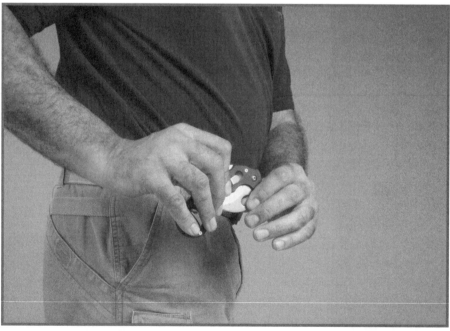

Once cleared from the carry position, the support hand moves to execute a safe open by separating blade from handle.

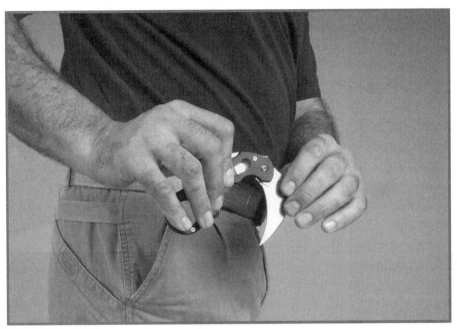

Using the support hand move blade from unlocked to locked position.

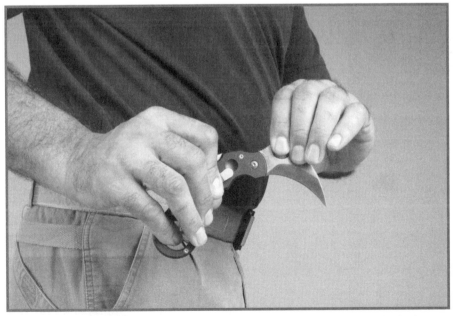

Continue to move toward the locked blade position until blade motion stops. This is the indication that the blade has moved as far as possible and should be now locked into place.

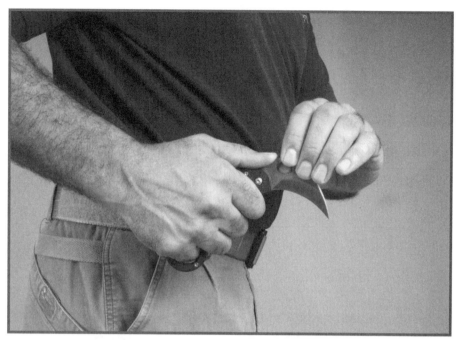

*Utilizing both visual and tactile confirmation, ensure
that the blade is in fact in the locked position.*

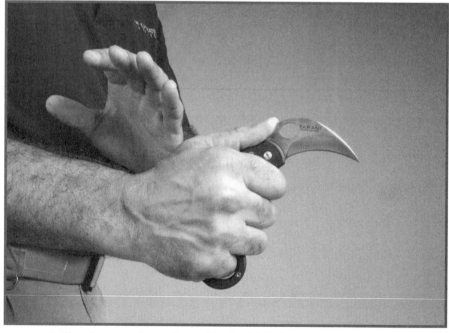

*Following confirmation of locked blade position, you may
then move to the ready position of your choice.*

The remaining alternate method of rapid deployment of the folding curved blade results in the blade facing downward or "reverse" grip. The advantages are that it is a little bit quicker to mount. However, the down side is that it's not as powerful a grip as the blade facing forward tip up.

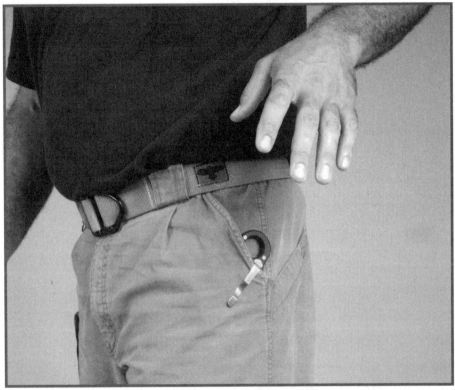

Starting from dominant hand side (strong side) in the example left pocket carry, begin with your hand above the pocket line.

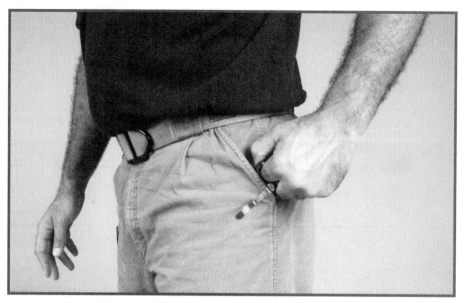

Inserting your forefinger directly into the safety ring, establish a firm and positive grip with a closed fist supporting the index finger. Note that you will NOT be able to mount the safety ring all the way through with the index finger from this initial position. This is the reason why all fingers are needed for grip support during deployment.

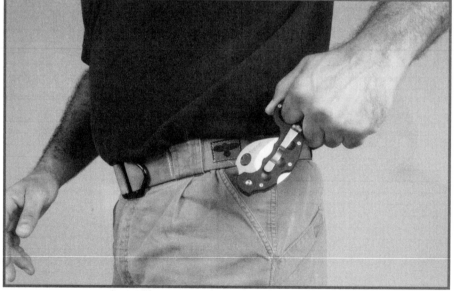

Upon mounting the index finder utilizing the safety ring clear the folding curved blade from it carry position.

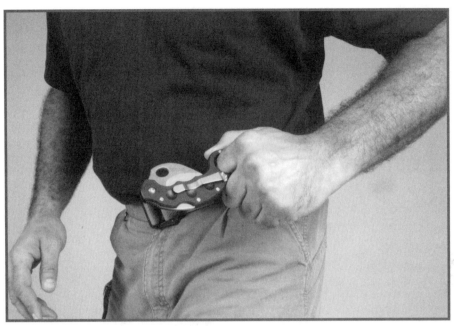

*Initiating a forceful snap of the wrist begins to loosen the blade
and initiate centrifugal force engaging the pivot screw.*

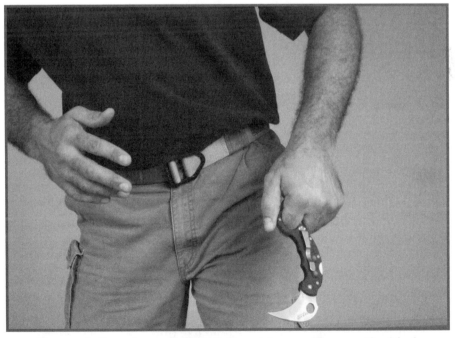

*If enough force is applied centrifugal force will cause the blade
to snap rapidly into the locked position.*

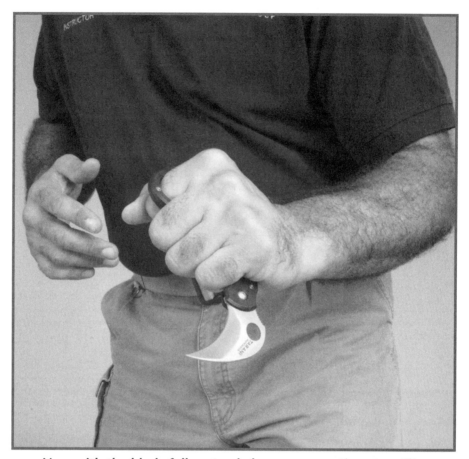

Now with the blade fully extended you may continue to utilize the blade in the extended position or take the extra second to spin it back into a more stable retracted position. Note the position of the support hand—behind and away from the blade.

As an instructor teaching throughout the professional training community for the past two decades, I am often asked to demonstrate opening a curved folding blade with the Emerson Wave ®. Due to the unique nature of the Wave ® and the position of the safety ring, an opening sequence might look something like this:

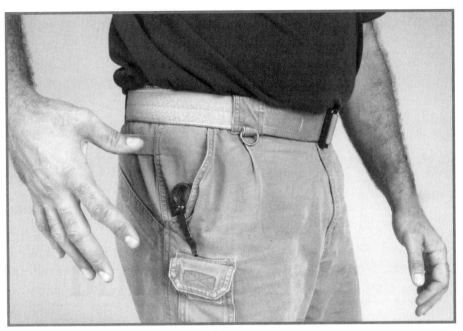

Reach for the strong side carry position.

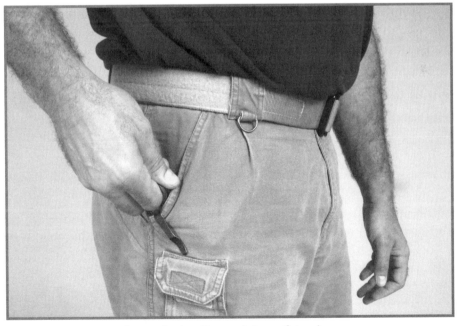

Insert index finger into safety ring.

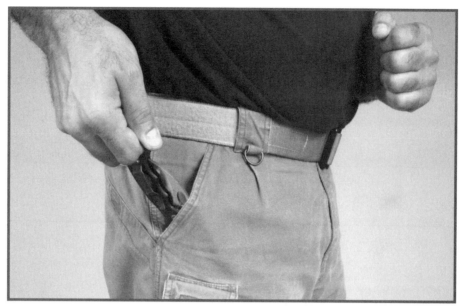

Press forward against the Wave device causing it to catch the forward part of the garment pocket and using that connection between material and Wave device to initiate open of the blade.

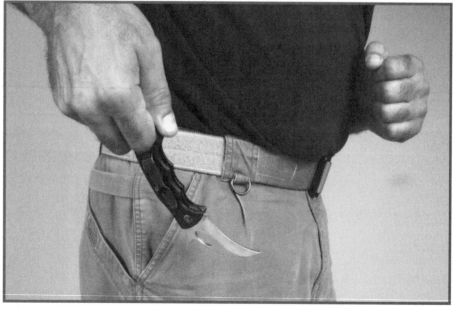

Continuing to press forward (provided that your garment material did in fact "catch the Wave") which should result in a full and complete locking of the folding curved blade.

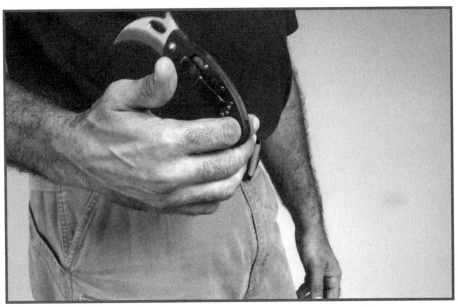

Following the blade locked in the open position, it is now feasible to change grips from extended to retracted by spinning as per above.

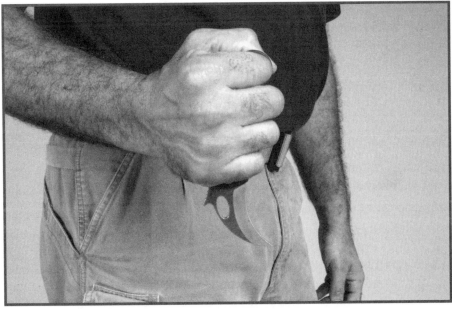

Ultimately you want to keep your support hand behind the strong hand and of course away from the tip and edged of the curved blade.

Now that we've covered the fundamentals of basic history, the differences between fixed and folding, curved blade selection, functional parts, carry, locking, unlocking, grips and mounts, deployment and rapid deployment, how can all of this be put together in such a manner as to be utilized for personal safety?

Part II
Personal Safety

PERSONAL DEFENSE

In this section, our focus of study will be placed squarely on the usage of the curved blade as it is applied to personal safety and defense.

The first question that comes to mind is, "Exactly what is personal safety?" The answer varies based on perspective, but a general rule of thumb is when you are legitimately in fear for your life or loss of limb (severe bodily injury) for yourself or those who may be with you such as family or friends. When are you *allowed* to defend yourself? In most cases, the real answer is when you perceive a realistic threat.

Keep in mind that (given sufficient reaction time and enough space) you always have the option to not engage with the threat and simply run away. If you have the time and the space then this is always recommended as an optimal response to a threat and will be covered in greater detail later.

The curved blade—like any other knife, when used for personal protection can be utilized as an implement of opportunity (some police departments use the term "weapon of opportunity"). However, you need to thoroughly consider this critical aspect of personal defense. Sure you have the ability to rip the bad guy's throat out by the roots, but you will then be held liable for your actions by a court of law—both criminally and civilly. Unfortunately in our most-litigious society, this is a recurring nightmare scenario and we see time and time again how the criminal is "wronged." How many times have you seen on TV or heard on the news or read in the paper that some dirt bag broke into a poor family's house, was confronted by the rightfully defensive homeowner and then sued the victim and won!

There's an important item called the "Use of Force continuum" which is a measuring device utilized by the courts to determine "wrongful use of force" in police activities where use of force may be applied. In fact this measuring device is not restricted to law enforcement application; it applies to civilians as well. There are a number of different Use of Force models—each state has their own version and sometimes it can vary from city to city. The federal Use of Force continuum differs from agency to agency, but there's quite a bit of overlap between them and those of the individual states and just about all law enforcement agencies offer their own interpretation based on circumstances and case law. Use of Force specialists are mostly attorneys who work these kinds of cases on a regular basis.

Although not quite as rigid and binding as for law enforcement professionals (who unfortunately must adhere to an additional filter of departmental policy regarding use of force)—civilians are most certainly held liable for their actions with regards to use of force. A general rule of thumb is to at least match the use of force being applied to you and if justified you can escalate to the next level. Please check with your local law enforcement professionals for more accurate details on use of force.

Escalation to the next level of force is what gets most people in trouble. If you get caught in a life-or-death struggle and your curved blade is the only thing standing between you living or dying, you still need to find that balance of application and move only to that level of force necessary to objectively and reasonable stop the threat. However, if your life depends upon it then you may want to bone up on some useful curved blade technology.

The personal safety skills one can acquire with a curved blade are numerous. Additionally they are purposely divided into two categories of instruction. One category is the necessary Combative Concepts which are utilized to engage or disengage from a threat. The other is Hard Skills which is the actual physical application. You can think of the former as loading software onto your computer and the latter as the computer itself. No system of personal defense training is complete without both software and hardware. Let's take a look at the first half of our personal protection training utilizing the curved blade as a viable personal safety option.

COMBATIVE CONCEPTS

Mindset

Paramount to any interpersonal conflict is proper mindset. If it's the case that your philosophy may be that all people are loving caring individuals and that nobody out there in the world wants to harm you, then you will be brutally surprised, taken completely off balance and will suffer maximum casualties as a result of this mindset with regards to an attack on your person. If, on the other hand, your mindset is such that there are some bad folks out there both intent and capable of delivering debilitating beat down as well as death to their next victim, then at least you have a leg up on the sheep of our society.

The next layer in mindset is "what if." You ask yourself, "What if I come around that dark corner in the parking lot at night and there's some large athletic male somewhere between 21 and 28 who is intent on getting what he wants from me regardless of my reaction?" Without asking these "what if" scenario questions you are not open to at least formulating an optimal response if the scenario were to occur. How many times have you found yourself thinking about something else, or all wrapped up in your cell phone call as you're walking through a potentially hazardous area (bad part of town). This second consideration—most often referred to as "general awareness" is equally as important to your philosophy regarding interpersonal conflict.

Lastly, in order to be effective, you must have some kind of a plan. If the only things you know are what you see in the movies or you simply have no plan then you will be caught WAY behind the power curve and may never catch up.

In summary mindset is all about how you look at something—it's simply a point of view. You can choose to espouse any mindset you wish; however, in order to be effective in response to an actual threat, it is strongly recommended that you at least consider these three:

First and foremost keep the mindset that there are some bad folks out there both intent and capable of causing you harm—because (contrary to the liberal media) they are out there.

Second, if you find yourself in a bad part of town or in a dark alley or maybe even approached by a stranger, it's important to run "what if" scenarios in your mind to prepare you mentally (loading the software) to handle any situation that may erupt unexpectedly.

Last, but certainly not least, is to have a plan. If your state is one of the few that still honors the U.S. Constitution and your right as a citizen of this great and free republic to own and bear arms, then best case scenario is to apply for your concealed weapons carry permit and get trained to both carry and use a handgun for personal safety. If this is not possible for whatever reason, then you need to have a plan of action and movement; a part of that plan may be to consider carrying and training with a curved blade.

Range, Position, Mobility

The three most important elements in any altercation are Range, Position and Mobility. It is of critical importance that you take control of all three of these elements. The degree to which you lose control of any one or more of these is to the degree to which you have given control of them to your adversary.

Let's take a look at each one individually starting with range. What is meant by range is simply distance, that is, how far away are you physically located from your attacker. There are only two ranges: Non-Contact Range (NCR) and Contact Range (CR). NCR is that range where he cannot reach you in any way. If you end up in a personal altercation then this is the best range to be at as it gives you the greatest number of options which will be covered in more detail later. CR is the range where you are at "bad breath distance" from your attacker where he can reach out with a knife, impact weapon or even his bare hands and deliver damage or possibly death to your person—this is by far the uglier of the two ranges of personal combat.

The second critical element is position. Position is the location of your body relative to your attacker. You might be behind him, or maybe he is behind you. Perhaps you are standing in front of him, or maybe he is off to the side of your body. Basically there are 360 degrees on the compass and you can be attacked from any one of these by a single individual as well as by multiple attackers. The safest position is to be either behind your attacker at contact range or simply out of range (NCR) from any physical contact.

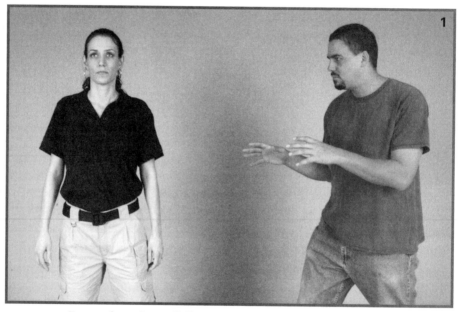

Examples of possibility of an attack from any angle.

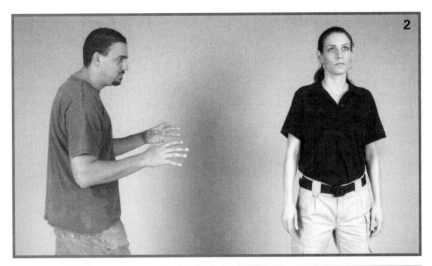

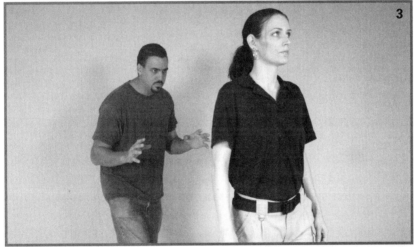

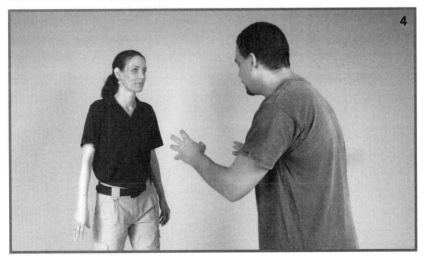

The final element is mobility. As we are all well aware a moving target is more difficult to hit than a stationary target. If you find yourself locked on your heels and immobilized, this is a less than optimal mobility scenario. You need to get moving. Start moving. DO NOT remain stationary! Continue to walk in an alternate direction, continue to create space and continue to keep him off balance trying to catch up to you while you formulate your next plan of action on the run. The instant you remain stationary is the same time you give up your effective response options.

Reactionary Gap

In addition to the three critical elements of controlling any fight (range, position and mobility) there are certain relationships between these elements that can be utilized as combative concepts (software) to keep your opponent off balance and trying to catch up to you. One of the most important of these is called a Reactionary Gap. Similar to the great sport of American football where a short yardage pass/run play is executed in less time than a long yardage pass/run play, there is a time/space relationship in combat that states that the less space between you and the assailant as his attack begins, the less time you have to react to that attack. If less space equals less reaction time, then the converse is also true: more space equals more reaction time. Additionally known as time/space (by the training industry experts), if you know what you're doing, the Reactionary Gap can be effectively used against your adversary.

Liability Gap

Another combative relationship is what is commonly referred to as the Liability Gap. Given the time/space relationship above, it's important to keep in mind that the closer he gets to you (less distance—which also means less reaction time) the greater your potential for personal injury. Let's say he's coming at you with a sharp knife swinging wildly. If you get out of the way at NCR of course you will sustain no injuries, but the second he can make contact with your fingers now you're going to need a band-aid. The deeper he moves into CR the higher your scale of injury. Instead of fingers he moves closer and cuts your wrist or biceps and if he moves in even closer (again less space and less time to react) he can have access to your throat and eyes and that's a pretty bad scenario because you have allowed the altercation to degenerate to a contact range engagement while remaining immobile and in terrible position.

SAFEST OPTION

The safest option in any personal conflict is to not be there—simple as that. If you have the option to drop what you're doing and get the heck out of Dodge, then that's your safest option. Why? Let's take a look at the factors involved. If you turn heels and run away you've successfully created more space which in turn creates more reaction time and additionally puts you in a position of advantage as well as being fully mobile. You have effectively increased the reactionary gap and simultaneously lowered your potential for personal injury. So, where's the downside to all this? There isn't one. Given all of the above when you make the decision to disengage from the threat and vacate the area, then you can check off all the boxes and although maybe a little shaken up psychologically after something like that, you remain home free and without personal injury.

CYCLES OF ACTION

Everything in our lives is based on cycles of action. Nature provides us the best example of this every day with the rising and setting sun. During the rotation of the Earth in orbit around the sun, seasons change and cycle back the following year. Everything is a cycle. Take the simple act of opening a door. You walk up to the door, you turn the knob, you walk through the door and the cycle repeats itself again when you come up to another door. If you're into firearms training, you will note that in the case of semi-automatic pistols that a round is cycled into the chamber, fired and after extraction and ejection of the remaining casing (provided you're using a fully loaded magazine) another round is cycled into battery. We can take and effectively apply this cycle of action concept to personal safety and defense in the event of interpersonal conflict.

OODA

One of the most famous cycles of action in the professional training community is the OODA cycle. This stands for Observe, Orient, Decide and Act. Each of these steps is repeated sequentially and is additionally one of the most important (if not THE most important) cycle of action in personal combat.

How it works is very simple. Let's say it's late at night and you're walking back to your car from the ATM machine and you see someone (a shady character) approaching you—you *observe* a potential threat. The next step in the OODA cycle is to *orient* to this potential threat. As part of that orientation step in the cycle, you ask yourself such questions as how far away is he from me? Where (what direction) is he coming from? Does he have any weapons in his hands? Next, based on the answers to those questions you then need to make a *decision*—do I stay and confront this threat or do I disengage and avoid it? Based on that decision you then follow through and *act* upon it. Then when that shady character starts to turn and follow you, the old OODA cycle starts all over again, you *observe* that he has changed his direction, you *orient* to the new set of circumstances, you then make a *decision* based on that orientation and finally you take *action* based squarely on that decision.

Deployment Decision

In the event of an attack on your person by an adversary or adversaries, there are an infinite number of responses. Looking at every single aspect of the scenario such as: Is he armed? Are you armed? Are there other people around? Is it dark or light? Are you in a confined area or is there open space? Is he already at Contact Range or are you still at Non-Contact Range? Does he have capability and intent to inflict severe bodily injury or death? All of these and many more variables contribute to the very difficult decision of whether to stay and engage the threat or to simply take the safest option and exit.

If there is little or no time to disengage, or react, or to change range or change position or maintain mobility and you have no other remaining options other than to stand there and accept severe bodily injury or death, (and you happen to be carrying your folding curved blade), then you may need to make that decision to deploy. If you have NO OTHER options and as a matter of self-preservation or the life and limb of another, you have made the decision to deploy, then what are your options with the curved blade as a matter of physical skills?

HARD SKILLS

Fighting Platform

If you are in the military and you want to set up a strong line of defense against the enemy, it's critical that personnel be well-trained, well-equipped and have a solid foundation or base established from which to begin the effort. This same principle applies to a professional boxer. To ensure success, he must be well-trained, be well-versed in his strategy (have a plan) and be able to both attack and defend from a stable "base." In the case of interpersonal conflict, a strong base simply means "stance" or how you present yourself in the event that you may need to defend yourself from that position—this is also referred to as a "stable base" or "fighting platform." Certain training academies use the term "stable fighting platform" to describe the initial (and optimal) position (stance) from which to deliver an effective personal defense.

A stable fighting platform can be achieved by simply placing your feet about shoulder width apart and have your toes facing toward the threat. Your hands should be up in preparation to defend against an attack. Lastly, and what most folks forget especially in the heat of battle, is to face your threat. Always be facing in the direction of the threat and constantly monitoring (observing) the change in conditions of your threat such as distance (range), your position relative to your threat and of course if you are mobile or stationary. There are a number of factors including Reactionary Gap and Liability Gap considerations, but all of these combative concepts—as valuable as they are—won't do you any good if you don't start with a stable Fighting Platform.

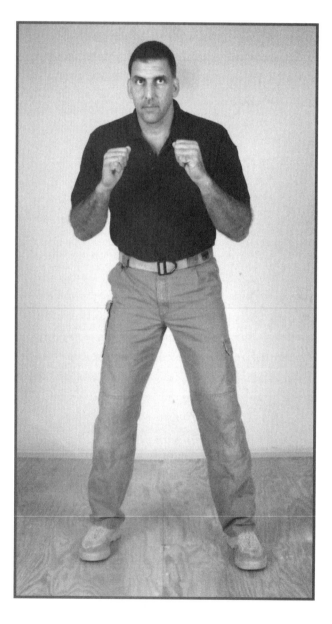

Feet should be at least shoulder width apart, toes facing down range, hands up and eyes on your threat.

In the event of an attack it is necessary to run rapidly through your OODA cycle and when it comes time to act, the first order of business is to establish a stable fighting platform. The quicker you get into that platform the better chance you have of effectively defending your position.

A training partner of mine has a great one-liner that exactly fits this combative concept. "You need to go from zero to hero." In the blink of an eye you must have the capability to go from hands below your belt, or in your pocket or doing something else to an immediate position of defense including your entire body turned facing the threat with feet shoulder width apart (or greater), hands up above your waistline and ready to fight. All of this must happen in less than a second.

Here's a simple drill you can run to train getting into this stable fighting platform:

Stand facing a mirror relaxed with your hands in your pockets and maybe just leaning off to one side on one foot. Then on the next audio cue you hear from your environment (slamming car door, baby crying, window opening, someone yelling from across the street, phone ringing, etc.) immediately move from your relaxed (soft) body posture, to a stable fighting platform as per above. Utilizing audio cues from your environment ties you into the dynamics of real-world response.

Posturing

Snapping into a stable fighting platform and then rapidly deploying your curved blade would give anyone a start—especially your attacker. The curved blade is a relatively "new" personal safety implement and not many bad guys have had much exposure to this tool as it is not as mainstream as a conventional straight blade.

Seeing a would-be victim snap into a stable fighting platform and rapidly deploy a curved blade will certainly get the attention of your assailant. It may very well cause him to stand there for a second running his own OODA cycle in order to make sense out of what just happened. While he's thinking about it, this is your cue to take the safest option: get out of there. Disengage from the threat and in so doing significantly reduce the odds on sustaining any personal injury. You may in fact have the upper hand in this situation and are so emotional about it that you may want to engage this attacker, but remember the criminal and then civil liabilities involved, where would your actions place you on the scale of injury and where would they place your attacker?

The safest action is to create distance. All real-world operators live by the same rule—in distance there is safety. Distance buys you time, which buys you opportunity to think more clearly and be able to evaluate your condition and then make a decision and then act on that decision. There is no close second. This is why it is referred to as the safest option. Disengaging from a threat will reduce your scale of injury, increase your personal safety and decrease your personal liability (criminal and civil).

Screaming and yelling and bringing attention to yourself in public is a VERY good idea, this way people can clearly see that you are in fear for your life (some attorneys recommend you even yell out the phrase—"I am in fear for my life!")

The bottom line here is that the simple act of posturing may be good enough to solve the problem.

Keep Aways

In the event that screaming, drawing attention and posturing are not working, you even try to disengage yet the assailant persists in his attack. In this scenario, having exhausted the first few layers of the use of force continuum (posturing, verbalizing, attempting to flee) it is clearly apparent that you have only two remaining personal safety options— allow yourself to become a victim (generally considered less than optimal) or keep this assailant away from you.

You've already tried posturing (moving to a stable fighting platform and then rapidly deploying your curved blade) and that didn't have any effect. The attacker continues to move toward you clearly demonstrating capability and intent to inflict serious bodily injury and perhaps even death. What are some additional options next in line on the use of force continuum?

Immediately moving to a stable fighting platform a simple yet effective means of keeping the attacker away from your body is to utilize your already rapidly deployed curved blade at NCR. Skillfully swing it in front of him in an effort to dissuade him from any further attack on your person. Remember that at this stage in the attack you are still at a relatively safe distance at non-contact range and with a wider reactionary gap this allows you more options and time to formulate a plan. The safest option here is to make space and utilize this non-contact range to disengage from your threat.

There are three defensive movement patterns of the blade which have been passed down to us through the centuries by the masters of personal safety. They are:

Forehand and Backhand

Side to side

Circular

Let's take a look at each of these in closer detail. One of your options in attempting to keep the attacker away from you is to swing the blade in a forehand and backhand movement similar to swinging a tennis racquet forehand and backhand while hitting the ball back over the net, use that analogy to guide your hand placement.

Keep Away 1

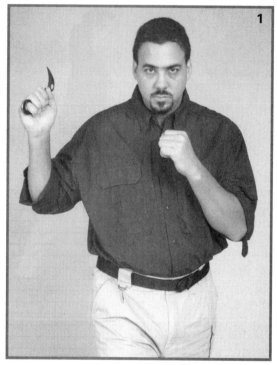

Beginning from the high-open and ready position, keep both hands up and remain in a stable fighting platform facing your threat.

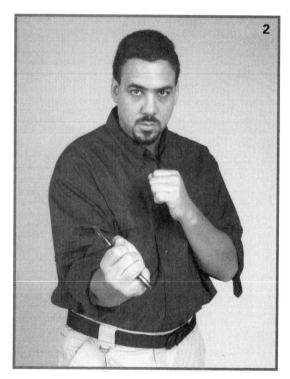

Strike from the high open position along a diagonal line of movement keeping the blade between you and your attacker.

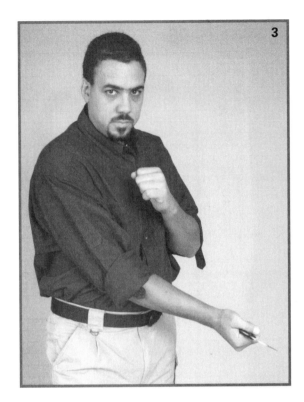

Continuing your swing, move the blade past the center of your body between yourself and the attacker thus completing the forehand strike.

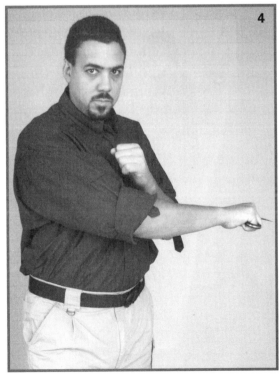

Immediately following completion of the forehand defensive strike pattern, begin the backhand defensive strike pattern by raising the blade to the high closed ready position.

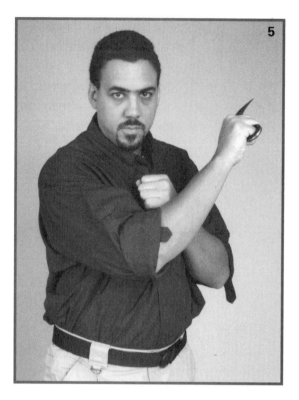

Starting from the high closed position, maintain a stable fighting platform.

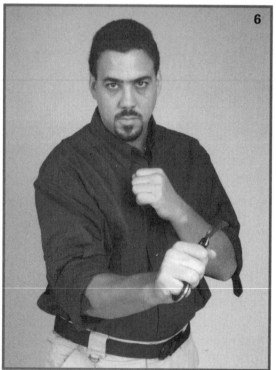

Continuing to move the blade in downward cutting motion, keep a safe distance between yourself and the attacker.

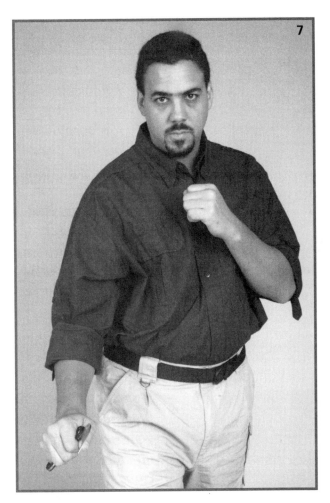

Completing the backhand defensive strike pattern it may be necessary to begin again at the high open ready position and repeat as necessary until the situation allows you the safest option— get the heck out of Dodge.

Keep Away 2

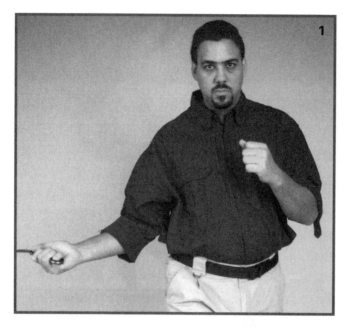

Starting from palm up grip mount in the low open ready position, begin to swing the blade horizontally across the center of your body in the space between yourself and the attacker.

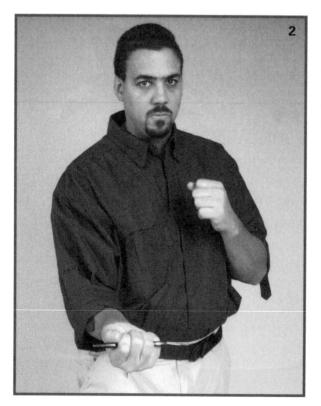

Maintaining palm up position keep your support hand up high for both counter-balance as well as additional high line protection.

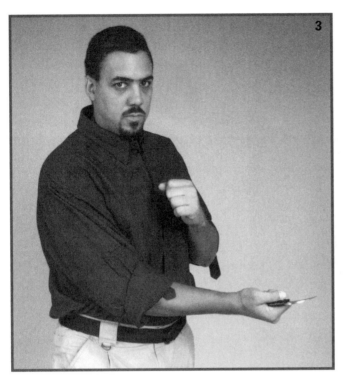

Complete the first horizontal pattern by moving the blade completely past your center line, maintaining a palm up grip mount.

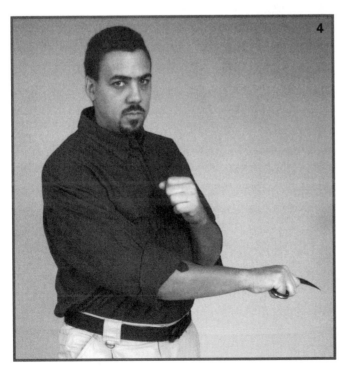

Now past center it's time to go back the other way following along that exact same horizontal defensive strike path. At this time, turn your hand to the palm down position.

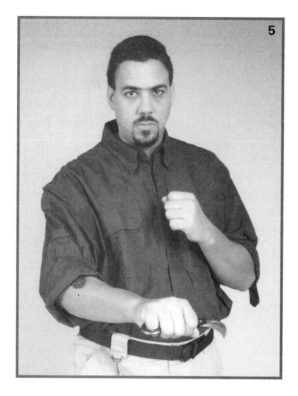

Continuing from the palm down position move the blade along that same horizontal line between yourself and the attacker.

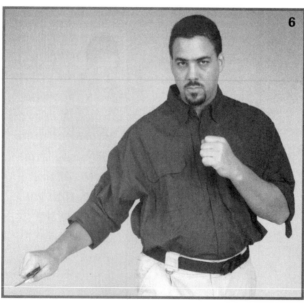

Ending in the palm down position past your center line effectively occupying the space between yourself and the attacker with a rapidly moving curved blade. From here it may be necessary to begin the entire cycle over again in order to move toward the safest option—get the heck out of Dodge.

Keep Away 3

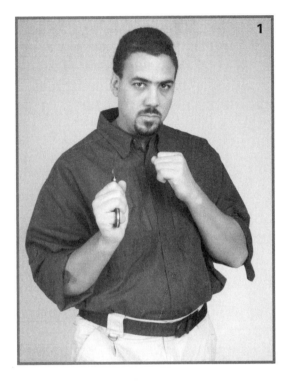

Beginning with both hands up and with the blade in the low guard ready position, maintain a stable fighting platform and remain facing the threat.

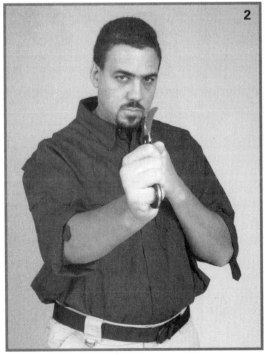

Push the blade out in front of you directly along a straight vertical line along the center of your body between yourself and the attacker.

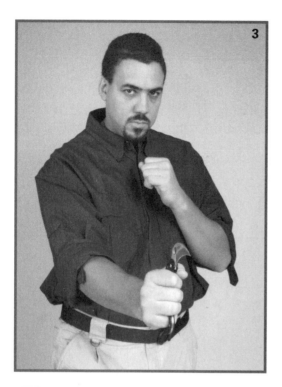

Continuing in a circular motion move to the fullest radius of that circle (full extension of your blade arm), allowing for maximum space between you and your attacker.

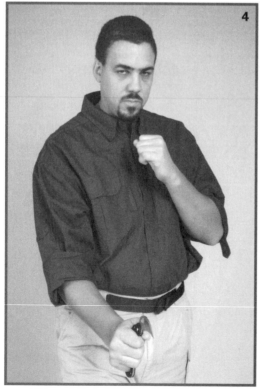

Now at the bottom of the circular patter begin to retract the blade along that same line of defensive strike pattern back toward your body.

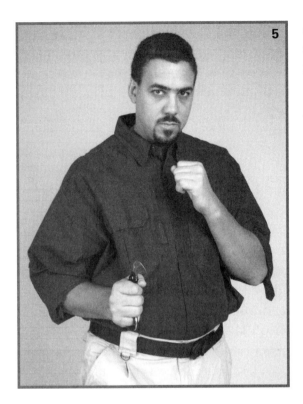

Now at the back of the circle, continue to move the blade upward along the same line back to your original position.

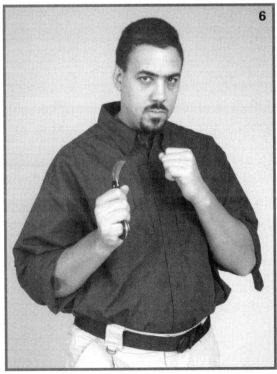

Completing the full circle puts you right back where you started and able to execute the exact same sequence again if needed or multiple times after that if needed to move toward the safest option—get the heck out of Dodge.

The whole purpose of the keep aways is to provide a temporary safety barrier between yourself and the attacker for a brief moment of time to allow you range, position and mobility to move to the safest option. Swing, swing, swing and run away!!!

Primary Skills

It's important to look at the personal defense process from a wider angle. First, an attack was initiated at non-contact range and you responded initially by verbal commands (or yelling) while trying to physically disengage but that didn't work. You then went into a stable fighting platform, rapidly deployed your curved blade and tried posturing and that didn't work. The attacker continued to close distance on your position (but still at non-contact range) so you tried any one (or all) of the keep-aways but to no avail. The attacker kept moving forward into your space and in fact closed from non-contact to the dangerous contact range, further reducing the reactionary gap and increasing your potential for personal injury. You exhausted all options along the use-of-force continuum—now what? Everything you threw at him is just not cutting the mustard and he's still coming at you, so what's Plan B?

In the event the keep away (your last line of defense at non-contact range) fails, there are a number of defensive movements that can be accomplished with the curved blade at contact range. The intent here is to utilize both combative concepts (software) and technique (hard skills) in such a manner as to place you in a position of advantage so that you may move to the safest option.

Given that the conflict has now closed in to the dangerous contact range, it is critical to apply effective technique rapidly and decisively. With the curved blade already deployed and with your body already in motion, as well as in a stable fighting platform, it is possible to utilize the outside edge, inside edge (hooking from both the retracted and extended positions), standard grip, tip and point or any combination of the above.

Outside Edge

Starting with the outside edge of the curved blade, there are a number of options which can be applied in personal defense. First it's important to be familiar with your equipment before deciding which technique to utilize. Also, it may be the case that your set of dynamic circumstances (constantly changing range, position, etc.) may also dictate what techniques remain viable.

As previously covered, if you happen to be holding a fixed curved blade there are only two blade configurations—the outside edge is sharpened (double edged) or it is not. If it is a folding curved blade then there is only one option and that is a single edge located only on the inside of the blade with a false edge along the outside. Either way, if you happen to strike exposed human flesh with the outside edge regardless of configuration this will cause a reaction.

Just to be clear, a strike with a false edge may cause some reaction to your attacker in the heat of close quarter battle, but a strike with a sharp outside edge may cause even more of a reaction. Either way, striking with the outside edge is a tremendous deterrent to a threat intent on continued attack against you at contact range.

To become familiar with utilizing the outside edge, there's an excellent training drill that doesn't require more than a plastic or aluminum training blade (you can even use a pair of scissors if you do not have a training blade) and a training partner. Try this drill and see if it fits into your tool kit:

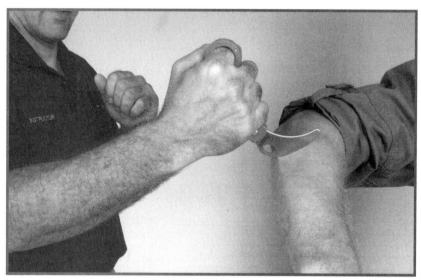

Gripping the curved training blade in the retracted blade down configuration and maintaining a vertical grip mount, apply a downward strike on your training partner's extended forearm (held in a horizontal position) in a slow and controlled manner so as to develop familiarization with the outside edge using a vertical grip.

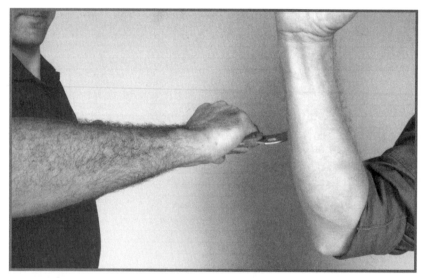

Gripping the curved training blade in the retracted blade down configuration and maintaining a palm down grip mount, apply a horizontal strike on your training partner's extended forearm (held in a vertical position) in a slow and controlled manner so as to develop familiarization with the outside edge using a palm downward grip.

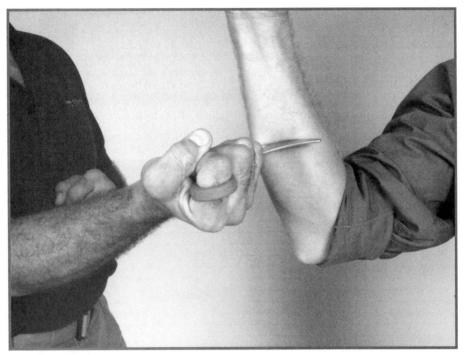

*Gripping the curved training blade in the retracted blade down
configuration and maintaining a palm up grip mount,
apply a horizontal strike on your training partner's extended
forearm (held in a vertical position) in a slow and controlled
manner so as to develop familiarization with the
outside edge using a palm upward grip.*

The next level up in the usage of the curved blade is application
of the inside edge or the hook. The hook can be applied in any one of
three positions: reverse grip (blade pointing downward) retracted, reverse
grip (blade pointing downward) extended and standard grip.

Application of the inside edge (more so than the outside edge)
against exposed human flesh can cause irreparable damage and is not recommended unless you have made the conscious decision that this is a life
or death situation and you need to do what it takes to walk away from
the attack alive and in one piece.

Inside Edge / Hook (Retracted)

The curved blade can be held in a grip mount with the blade facing downward (reverse grip) and with the handle retracted into the hand for a positive grip. Training from this configuration can gain familiarization with defensive strike applications. The following drill is design to provide such a familiarization and with additional repetition eventual proficiency.

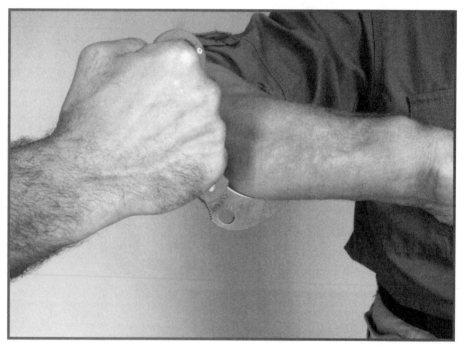

Gripping the curved training blade in the retracted blade down configuration and maintaining a vertical grip mount, apply an upward strike (hooking motion) against your training partner's extended forearm (held in a horizontal position) in a slow and controlled manner so as to develop familiarization with the inside edge using a vertical grip.

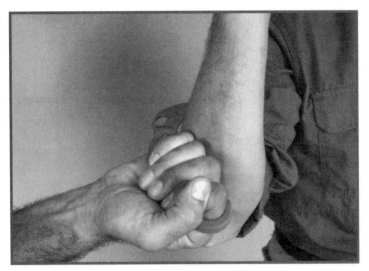

Gripping the curved training blade in the retracted blade down configuration and maintaining a palm up grip mount, apply a horizontal strike (hooking motion) on your training partner's extended forearm (held in a vertical position) in a slow and controlled manner so as to develop familiarization with the inside edge using a palm upward grip.

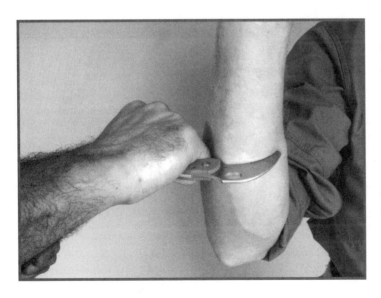

Gripping the curved training blade in the retracted blade down configuration and maintaining a palm down grip mount, apply a horizontal strike (hooking motion) on your training partner's extended forearm (held in a vertical position) in a slow and controlled manner so as to develop familiarization with the outside edge using a palm downward grip.

Inside Edge / Hook (Extended)

Although not as powerful a grip as the standard or the reverse grips, the extended grip is still capable of delivering debilitating strikes to soft targets on the human body. Remember that you can cut yourself shaving, so the application of a 3-inch curved piece of razor sharp hooked blade against an exposed body part or other soft target can cause devastating results.

The curved blade can be held in a grip mount with the blade fully extended by the safety ring and using the front and rear brakes for a positive grip. Training from this configuration can gain familiarization with defensive strike applications. The following drill is designed to provide such a familiarization and with additional repetition eventual proficiency.

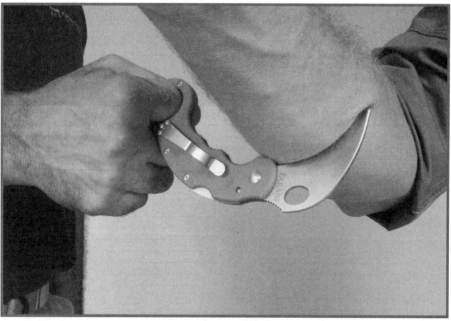

Gripping the curved training blade in the extended configuration and maintaining a vertical grip mount, apply an upward strike (hooking motion) against your training partner's extended forearm (held in a horizontal position) in a slow and controlled manner so as to develop familiarization with the extended inside edge using a vertical grip.

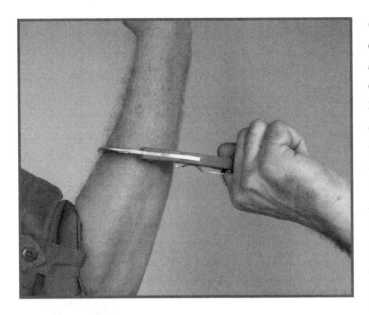

Gripping the curved training blade in the extended configuration and maintaining a palm up grip mount, apply a horizontal strike (hooking motion) on your training partner's extended forearm (held in a vertical position) in a slow and controlled manner so as to develop familiarization with the extended edge using a palm upward grip.

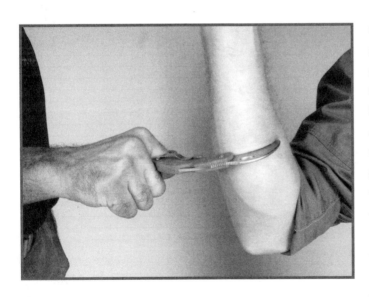

Gripping the curved training blade in the extended configuration and maintaining a palm down grip mount, apply a horizontal strike (hooking motion) on your training partner's extended forearm (held in a vertical position) in a slow and controlled manner so as to develop familiarization with the inside edge using a palm downward grip.

Standard Grip Hook

As covered earlier, the most powerful grip attainable with a curved blade utilizing the characteristic safety ring is the standard grip. This grip configuration allows maximum control, power and articulation of the blade while in motion during a violent and aggressive contact range attack. The advantages of this hand configuration are numerous; the blade cannot be disarmed (taken away from you in the fight), the blade is molded into your hand as an extension of your index finger, so where you point, you cut. The human body is already familiar with holding hammers, screwdrivers, forks, spatulas and other common items which allows a predisposed familiarity with this particular grip of the knife.

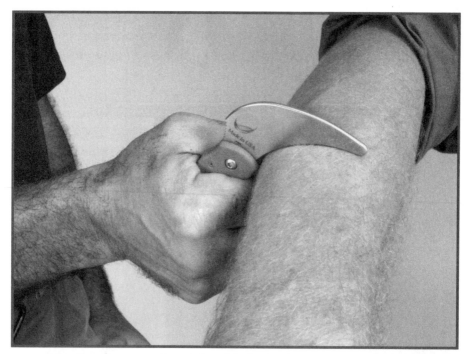

Gripping the curved training blade in the standard grip blade up configuration and maintaining a vertical grip mount, apply a downward strike (hooking motion) against your training partner's extended forearm (held in a horizontal position) in a slow and controlled manner so as to develop familiarization with the inside edge using a vertical grip.

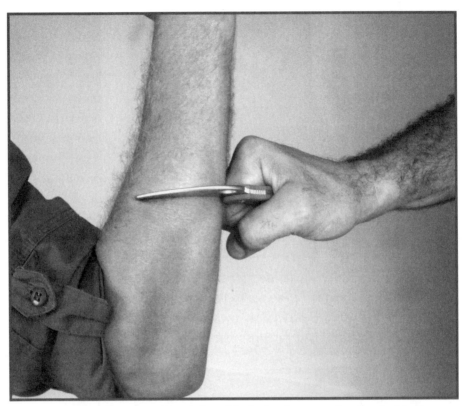

*Gripping the curved training blade in the standard grip blade
up configuration and maintaining a palm down grip mount,
apply a horizontal strike (hooking motion) on your training
partner's extended forearm (held in a vertical position) in a
slow and controlled manner so as to develop familiarization
with the inside edge using a palm downward grip.
Notice in this illustration the operator's thumb is
gripping his hand in a closed fist.*

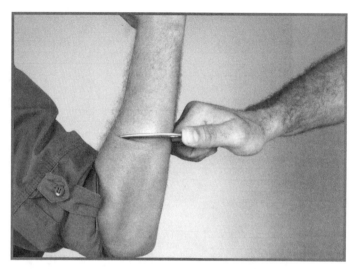

Gripping the curved training blade in the standard grip blade up configuration and maintaining a palm down grip mount, apply a horizontal strike (hooking motion) on your training partner's extended forearm (held in a vertical position) in a slow and controlled manner so as to develop familiarization with the inside edge using a palm downward grip. Notice in this illustration the operator's thumb is gripping the friction radius of the curved folding blade.

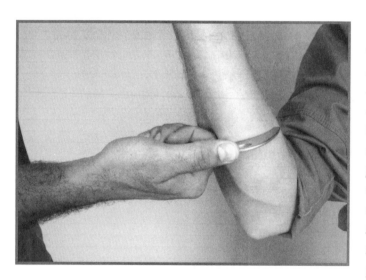

Gripping the curved training blade in the standard grip blade up configuration and maintaining a palm up grip mount, apply a horizontal strike (hooking motion) on your training partner's extended forearm (held in a vertical position) in a slow and controlled manner so as to develop familiarization with the inside edge using a palm upward grip.

Tip or Point

In a life or death struggle where you are literally in a fight for your life with your bare hands, you want to have as much effective technique as possible at your disposal to get yourself to the safest option. The next level up on the Use of Force continuum is application of the point or tip of the curved blade. Utilizing this part of the blade can be the most effective as a thrust with a blade is generally more effective than a slash. Additionally, this is the most familiar of all the blade movements to the novice as it is nothing more than application of a punch with a sharp object attached to your hand.

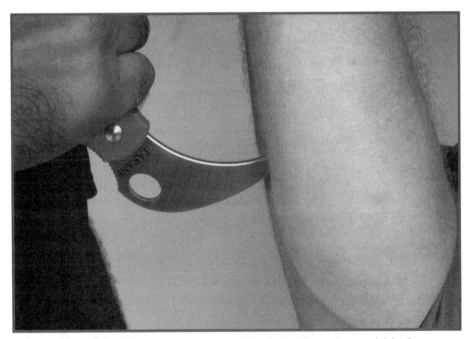

Gripping the curved training blade in the retracted blade down configuration and maintaining a vertical grip mount, apply an inward strike using the tip or point against your training partner's extended forearm (held in a horizontal position) in a slow and controlled manner so as to develop familiarization with the tip or point of the curved blade using a vertical grip.

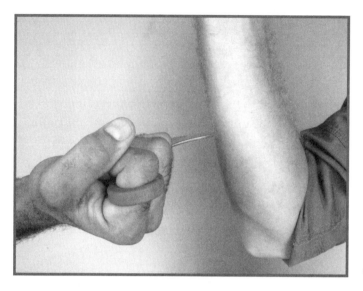

Gripping the curved training blade in the retracted blade down configuration and maintaining a palm up grip mount, apply an inward strike using the tip or point against your training partner's extended forearm (held in either a vertical or horizontal position) in a slow and controlled manner so as to develop familiarization with the tip or point of the curved blade using a palm up grip.

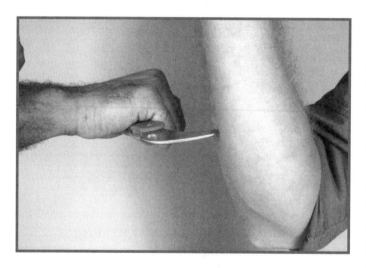

Gripping the curved training blade in the retracted blade down configuration and maintaining a palm down grip mount, apply an inward strike using the tip or point against your training partner's extended forearm (held in either a vertical or horizontal position) in a slow and controlled manner so as to develop familiarization with the tip or point of the curved blade using a palm down grip.

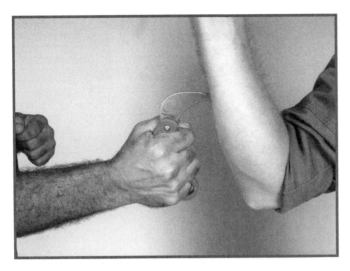

Gripping the curved training blade in the standard grip blade up configuration and maintaining a vertical grip mount, apply an inward strike using the tip or point against your training partner's extended forearm (held in a horizontal or vertical position) in a slow and controlled manner so as to develop familiarization with the tip or point of the curved blade using a vertical grip with the blade up.

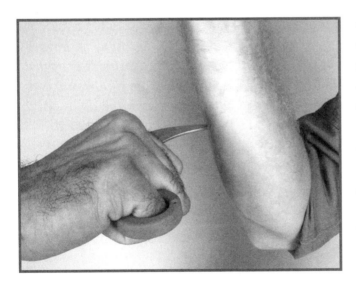

Gripping the curved training blade in the standard grip blade up configuration and maintaining a palm down grip mount, apply an inward strike using the tip or point against your training partner's extended forearm (held in a horizontal or vertical position) in a slow and controlled manner so as to develop familiarization with the tip or point of the curved blade using a palm down grip with the blade up.

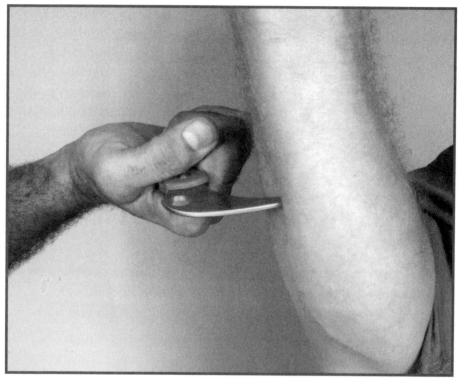

Gripping the curved training blade in the standard grip blade up configuration and maintaining a palm up grip mount, apply an inward strike using the tip or point against your training partner's extended forearm (held in a horizontal or vertical position) in a slow and controlled manner so as to develop familiarization with the tip or point of the curved blade using a palm up grip with the blade up.

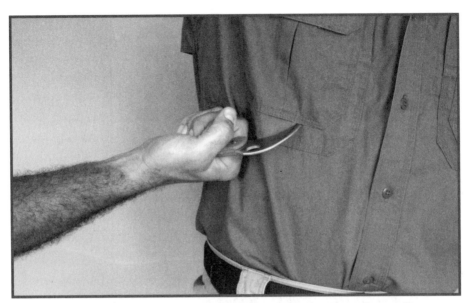

*In practical application (regardless of grip mount) a strike
with the tip (or any other part of the blade for that matter)
can be applied to any soft target of the human body.*

Combination Strikes

The very highest level of potential damage to your attacker is
combination or multiple striking. Combination strikes are nothing more
than a rapid succession of any or all of the above strikes applied to the
human body at contact range. Much like a professional boxer who delivers repetitive combination strikes to his opponent in the ring, a combination of strikes can generally cause an overload (similar to a short circuit
with electrical wires) of the nervous system and instantly persuade an
assailant to seek other activities.

Each of the above strikes isolated on their own can be very effective, but combining them in succession can be most devastating to an
attacker should they land successfully. Delivery of multiple applications
of the curved blade in succession to varying locations on the human
body is one of the most effective methods of employing your curved
blade to deter further attack and foster a safe option.

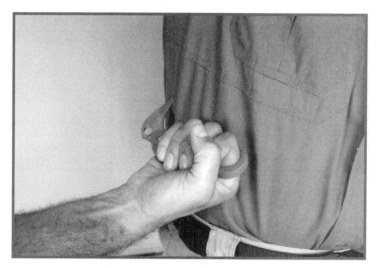

In practical application (regardless of grip mount) multiple or combination strikes with the tip (or any other part of the blade for that matter) can be applied to any soft target of the human body leading to effective short term results. Again, keep in mind that such application may be in response to an immediate threat to your life and personal safety.

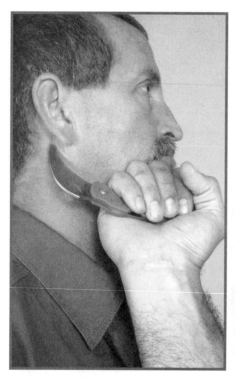 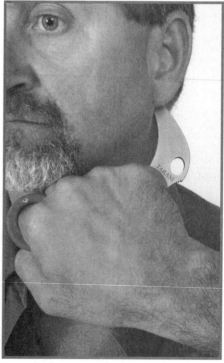

It is recommended that these training drills be repeated no less than ten, twenty or thirty times or even more to internalize the technique and develop familiarization and eventually proficiency.

Seated Position

In the real world a sudden and violent attack can occur at anytime and in any place. It may not always be the case that you are in the standing position. You could be caught in a seated position when the attack occurs and you may be required to take defensive measures while fighting for your survival from the seated position, perhaps in your car or at a park bench eating your lunch. It's a good practice to train for these different attack scenarios so that you are not taken by surprise and at least have some level of familiarity and proficiency with that particular defensive position.

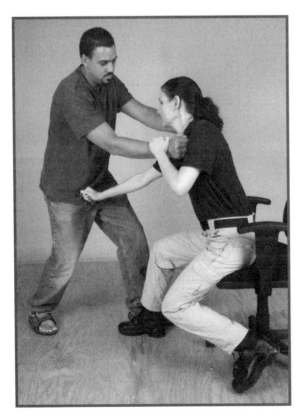

In the event that you may be attacked while in the seated position, it is still very important to maintain a stable fighting platform. Notice how the position of the feet and squaring off to the threat allow for effective placement of the blade against a soft target of the assailant's body.

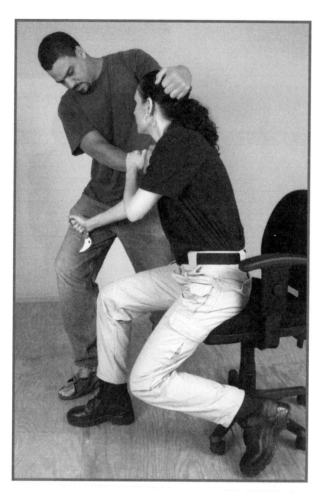

In this example the attacker is purposely not allowing the would-be victim to square off to him and gain maximum effective placement of the curved blade. Nonetheless, by maintaining a stable fighting platform, the defender is still able to immobilize one of her assailant's hands and based on proximity of blade to the attacker's body is able to deliver effective combination strikes to the legs causing him to back away in self preservation.

Armed with the personal survival tools of a good understanding of Combative Concepts (mindset, range, position, mobility, reactionary gap, liability gap, safest option, cycles of action, etc.), and Hard Skills such as the stable fighting platform, posturing, keep aways and primary defense skills, we can now focus our scope of study to the application of these tools in real world application.

PART III
DEFENSIVE TACTICS

DEFENSIVE TACTICS

Since the time you were a little kid most likely you were aware of the martial arts. In the local theater and on TV there are numerous cartoons, movies and television shows which dynamically illustrate the martial arts with cool moves, flying monkey kicks to the head, breaking bricks and wearing of heavy white cotton garments held together with a black belt. Thoughts like this go flying right out the window when it comes to an actual "in-your-face" real-world threat to your life. You are not in a gym or dojo, you're not barefoot, you're not warmed up for the big fight, you're not wearing gloves, you're not prepared for anything like this whatsoever and your mind is most likely anywhere but where it needs to be when you are unpleasantly surprised by an assailant.

The martial arts are exactly that—art. Like any art it takes from age eight to age eighty to gain true depth and understanding. No insult or slander intended here whatsoever or even implied against martial arts as I myself am a life-long devoted disciple to them. However, in the professional law enforcement, military and other federal agent training community there is very little or no time to spend on development of martial art skills. The only time available (and even that is always a bare minimum) is at best a handful of hours to learn some basic techniques and then you're in the field shortly thereafter with little or no follow-up training.

There are certain similarities between defensive tactics and the martial arts such as balance, form and function. Defensive tactics are, in fact, based on a foundational understanding of fundamental martial arts and the two are considered by most to be distant cousins. However, there are considerable differences between the two, the biggest difference being the ability for a trainee to pick up new and useful techniques with no prior background or training, and that the technique can only be a couple of gross-motor movements—no more than two steps, it must be executable in less than a second and a half, require zero memorization and must exactly fit into pre-existing academy training, department policy and also other component training such as firearms and other training requirements. These are often referred to not as "martial arts moves" but as "defensive tactics" or sometimes "active counter-measures."

For purposes of our scope of study in this manuscript the following techniques will be presented closer to the side of the defensive tactics than to the martial arts.

Anatomy of Attack

Any attack on your person at close quarters is comprised of critical elements such as physical location, body position, and time of day which have a direct bearing on the final outcome. Let's take a look at some of these important aspects and take a closer look at the anatomy of an attack situation.

Referencing physical location, these can include anything from an open parking lot, to a parking structure, or a secluded stairway, an ATM, a narrow hallway, running trail, or an unfamiliar part of the city. The assailant can be hiding under your car, can come leaping out from behind a bush or tree, from around the corner of a building, behind a mailbox or trash can, only your (and his) imagination is the limit.

Referencing body position, you can be approached by an attacker from any one of 360 degrees. Imagine yourself standing in the middle of an empty room with several doors and windows surrounding you along all four walls, now visualize one of these doors or windows opening and an assailant rapidly entering the room. If you can use your mind's eye to see the many different possibilities, this will provide a greater understanding in the first steps at being able to defend against such an attack.

Although you can be approached from all 360 degree angles of attack on your body, this complete circle can be broken down to only four positions—posterior, anterior, lateral left and lateral right—these are the DT descriptions, following are both static and scenario examples of the four cardinal directions of potential attack:

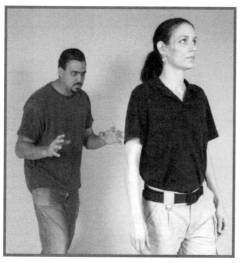

Posterior—from the back.

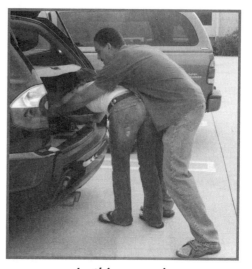

*In this example
the attacker approached
from behind—posterior.*

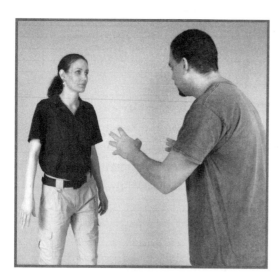

Anterior—from the front.

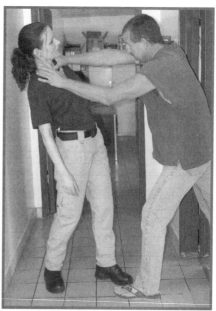

*In this example the
attacker approached
from the front—anterior.*

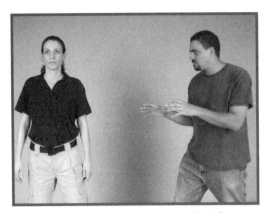

Lateral Left—On your left side.

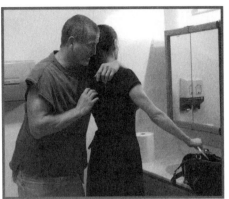

In this example the attacker approached from the lateral left.

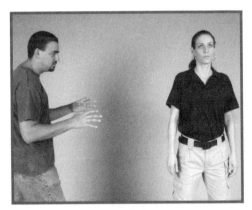

*Lateral Right—
On your right side.*

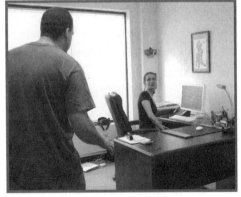

*In this example
the attacker approached
from the lateral right.*

Regarding time of day, a close quarters attack on your person can occur at any time morning, noon or night. The majority of attacks have been officially recorded by various state and federal law enforcement agencies, as occurring predominantly in low light conditions—that is mostly at night or in poorly-lit confined areas.

Finally, there are two key elements of any attack which favor the assailant. These are the surprise and the speed at which the attack occurs. The first of these, surprise, is always on the side of the attacker because the assailant will always decide when and how he will attack. The speed of the attack (the average attack occurs in less than 2.5 seconds) is simply action-reaction where the assailant has taken action and you are faced with no other option other than to react (which we'll go into later in greater depth) or simply remain a victim with no response at all. The choice is always yours.

Anatomy of Defense

Given all of the above: physical location, body position, time of day, etc, how can we best prepare to defend against an attack and further take control of that Action-Reaction power curve?

First, let's take a little break and review what we've got going here so far. Optimally you want to use your powers of observation, awareness, mindset and combative concepts training to maintain an awareness of your surroundings and counter-surveil the attacker prior to him getting within contact range. This way there's no need to move to a stable fighting platform or deploy, just continue to make distance and increase your range. Forewarned is forearmed.

The next level down is despite your awareness and counter-surveillance, he steps toward you at NCR, now due to applying your posturing technique he changes his mind and looks for a less difficult victim. You needed to deploy, but the situation still ended without confrontation.

The majority of your problems can be easily solved with all of the above. In fact, statistics support the fact that approximately 95% or greater of attack scenarios can be solved by simply keeping your wits about you maintaining a proper mindset and immediately demonstrating to the attacker that he's in for a difficult struggle should he continue to pursue his original attack plans. However, there is always that worst case scenario where you are forced to directly engage the threat. It may be the case that you find yourself physically in his "grasp" or "captured" so to speak, where he may have physically struck you or gained some type of physical control of your body. In this worse-case scenario you are forced to either engage the attacker directly or agree to become a victim. Again, the decision is completely up to you.

Agreeing to be a victim is considered less than optimal and not an option. You'd like to do the most sensible thing here and get the heck out of Dodge (which is in fact the overall safest option), but because you're at contact range now, there needs to be an interim step because now he's gone "hands on" and has posed an immediate threat to your life and/ or limbs.

Escapes

In some extreme cases you may be forced into a wooded area or into a van or into a closet, bathroom or other secluded area away from potential witnesses. Kidnapping, rape, murder, fill in the blank. It is critical to escape such a scenario.

As bad as this is, a number of optimal defenses are at your disposal. It's critical to first escape any physical immobilization that may be placed upon you by your attacker such as him grabbing your wrist or arm, pushing you to the ground, grabbing you by the throat or a piece of clothing and manipulating your body against your will in any manner. Once you've managed to escape his grasp you have become mobile, so the split second you gain mobility your next step is get the heck out of there as rapidly as possible. The two important steps are: escape his immediate grip and immediately escape from the danger area.

The following are some examples of physical grasps which clearly illustrate why being caught in such a disadvantageous position can place you at great risk leading to increased bodily injury or even death.

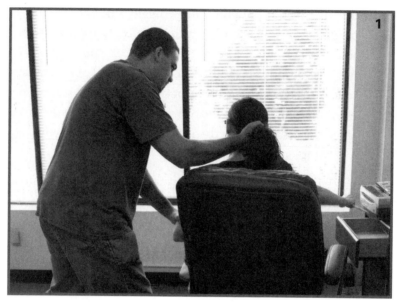

Hair and elbow grab.

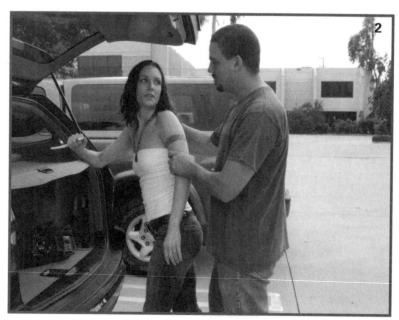

Arm and neck grab.

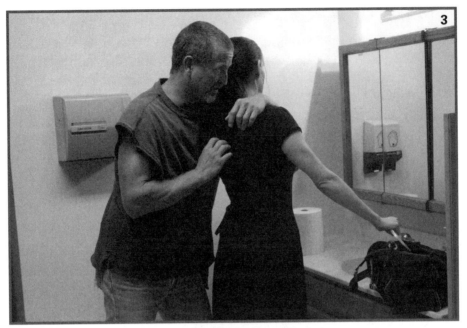

Throat and clothing grab.

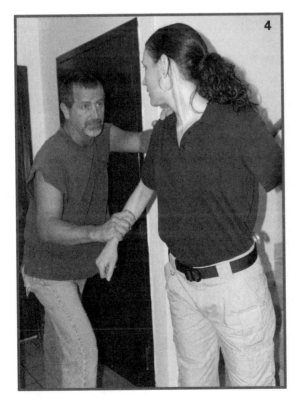

Wrist and shoulder grab.

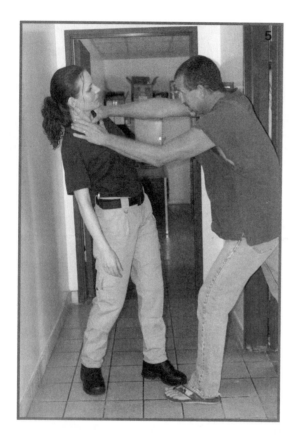

Throat grasp.

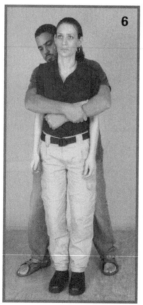

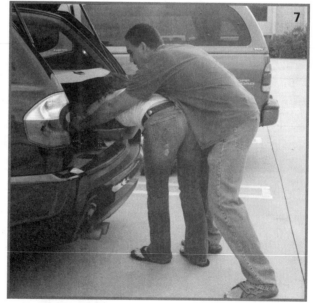

Double arm grabs.

Target Placement

It may be the case that you find yourself literally fighting for your life and limb. In this extreme condition and under such "fight-for-your-life" duress every action matters and every precious second counts. Again, the optimal solution is first become mobile and then use that mobility to vacate the danger area. However, step one is critical to your escape and given the extremity of the situation possibly to save your life.

If initial physical (unarmed) resistance fails to generate escape from such physical immobilization (grasp of your wrists, elbows, neck, hair, etc), it may be necessary to move to the next level of force objectively necessary to stop the threat. In such cases where you are certain that your situation looks as though it's going to further deteriorate to loss of life or limb, then your only remaining option is to move to deadly force.

Since you may be overpowered and overcome by the elements of both speed and surprise of the attack, you may literally find yourself in a physical struggle for your life. Of course you must check with your specific states laws, but in most states it is the opinion of the courts that use of deadly force to stop an immediate threat is justified in the event that your attacker possesses the means, intent and capability of causing severe bodily injury and/or death.

Should it be the case that you find yourself in such dire circumstances as the struggle for life or limb, and it is your perception that you are justified in the use of deadly force to stop this immediate threat, then your best option (should you not have access to a loaded firearm) is to deploy your curved blade. Once the curved blade is deployed, you can't just swing wildly in the air. You're at too close a range and you're lucky to even deploy the blade and he's too overcome by his intention to do bad things that you have no alternative but to immediately defend your position with the intention (and overall master plan) of getting out as quickly as possible.

OK, great. As circumstances would have it, you somehow managed (under extreme duress) to access and deploy your curved blade. Now what? What's the next step in getting free from his grasp, becoming mobile and vacating the threat area? The "A" answer is to deliver distractions (strikes to specific target areas) to your attacker's body with the intended result being that he will not want to continue his life-threatening attack and leave you alone.

There are a number of target areas on the human body so in order to simplify matters they can be divided into two categories: hard targets and soft targets.

Hard targets are the skeletal system of the body. Any bone of the arm, leg, or hip, for instance, or the head constitutes a hard target. While striking such hard targets with a sizable impact weapon can generate the desired response (the confrontation coming to an end), the curved blade is not optimal for application to hard targets.

Soft Targets

The remainder of the human body is comprised of soft targets: muscle and soft tissue such as the eyes, groin, and throat. These are the better choice of target when employing the curved blade. With barely only three inches, plus or minus, in blade length there is little or no chance of severing the abdominal aorta or inferior vena cava. However, the wrist (venal), the biceps (muscular) and the armpits are three "stages" to attack. Our scale of injury from earlier studies works both ways, the closer you get to his center mass (vital organs) the higher the scale of injury you will inflict upon your attacker. It's difficult to make these decisions on the fly, but suffice it to say that if you are in fact in danger of losing life or limb then your decisions at that time should be based accordingly. The neck, throat, inner arm, groin and inner thigh are all excellent target choices for attempting to stop a life-threatening attack with your curved blade. It makes no difference whether you deploy the curved blade in standard or reverse grip. Target acquisition is not hindered by either position as the following examples display in a variety of grips.

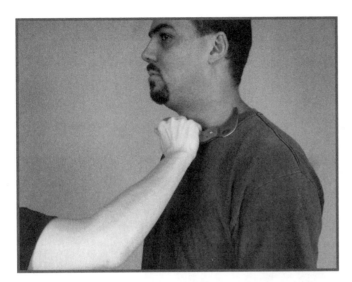

Soft targets are the preferred target with the curved blade. This example shows targeting of the neck and throat in the reverse grip, palm down position.

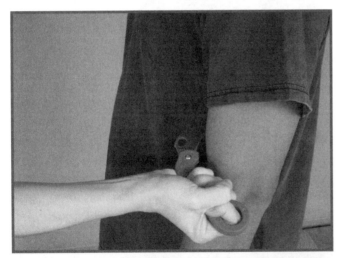

As seen in this example, soft targets include the inside of the assailant's arm, shown with the blade in the reverse grip with the palm both face up and down.

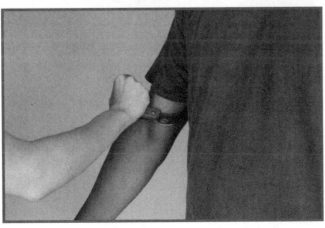

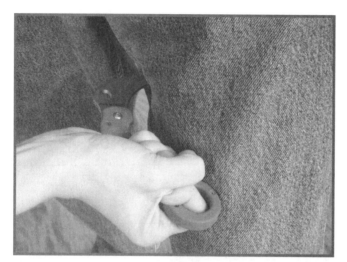

These three examples show additional soft targets for optimal use of the curved blade in the reverse grip: inner thigh and groin.

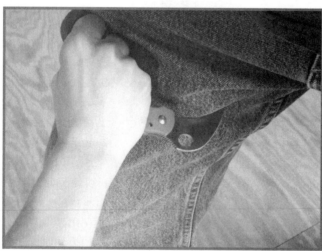

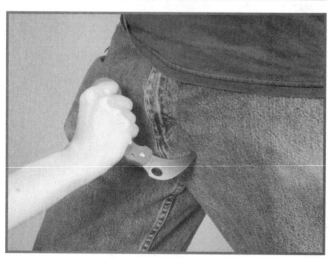

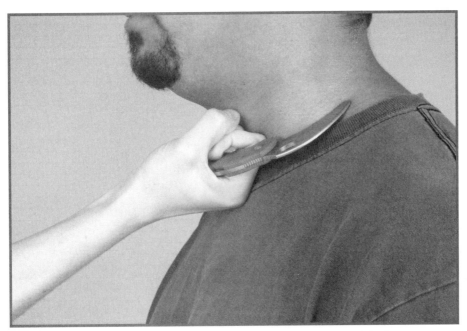

*Employing the strongest grip with the curved blade,
the standard grip, here are examples of acquiring
soft targets. Note the use of the curved blade once
again with both the palm up and palm down.*

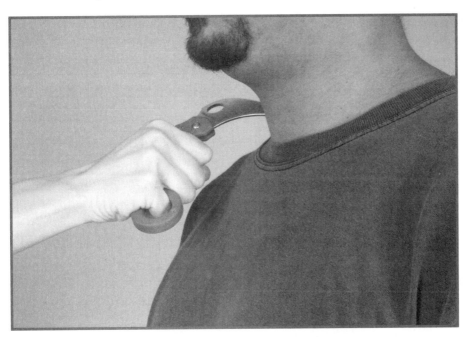

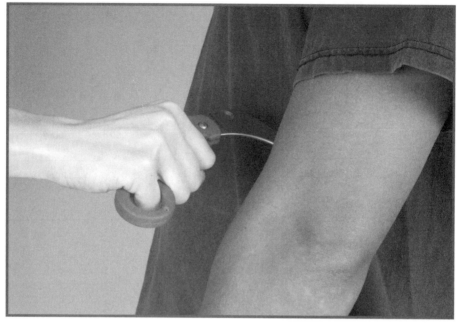

*Despite the different grip, target acquisition remains constant.
Here are examples of targeting the arm with a thrust. Again
the strikes are delivered both palm up and palm down.*

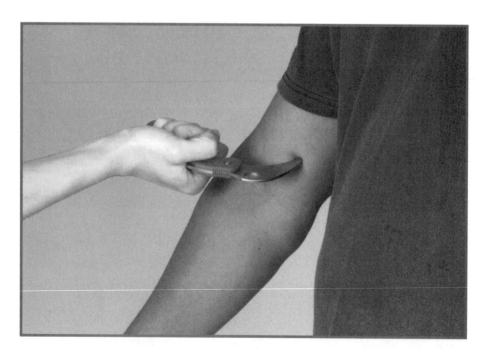

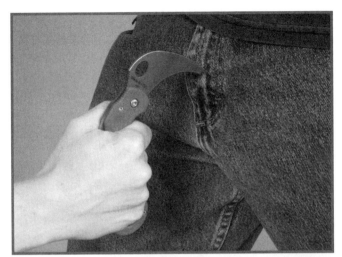

Similar to using the curved blade in the reverse grip, the groin and inner thigh are prime targets with the curved blade, this time in the standard grip.

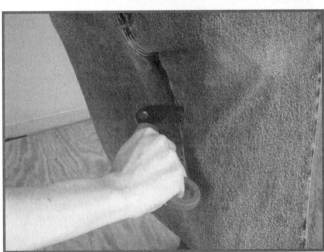

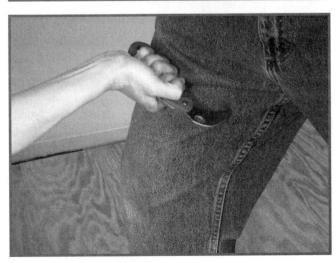

Regardless of attack approach, the worst case is that the attack goes down at Contact Range and it's so fast you didn't have time for Plan A, that is, Stage 1: Disable the nearest threatening target.

You may not even be able to reach a soft target based on your immediate physical condition. A hard target may be the only thing you can get. For example cutting the face (backed up by a hard skull) is not very high on the scale of injury, unless you make contact with the attacker's eyes, which are considered an optimal soft target as such a distraction can immediately impair the attacker's visual acuity, but it will certainly cause enough of a distraction and minor discomfort to possibly change your position and help you become mobile.

Immediately after gaining mobility, it is often advised to scream at the top of your lungs "Help, I'm in fear for my life!!" while bolting into an open, public area where you have removed yourself from the threat area and are in plain visibility of others in the vicinity.

Isolated Technique

Up to now we have covered quite a bit of material including curved blade selection, familiarization of blade parts, carry, grips and mounts, ready positions, rapid deployment, combative concepts, fighting platform, posturing, and other primary or "isolated" skills.

In preparation for practical application, the next step in our study is to combine these basics or "primary skills" in order to execute isolated technique. Only after gaining a comfort level in familiarization with isolated technique can we then move on to practical application of these techniques in dynamic scenarios.

In the following seven common examples of personal attack, it is assumed that the "victim" remained unaware of their surroundings (condition white) and was subsequently caught off guard by the attacker. With no other options remaining, the defender has the choice of remaining immobilized (a victim and at the mercy of the attacker) or taking control of the fight and as per above: 1. escape—become mobile (freed from the initial attack) and then, 2. rapidly move away from the threat area. It is also assumed throughout these isolated sequences, that the defender has access to their curved blade and was able to rapidly deploy in defense against a surprise attack.

Left Side Attack—Wrist Grab Escape Sequence

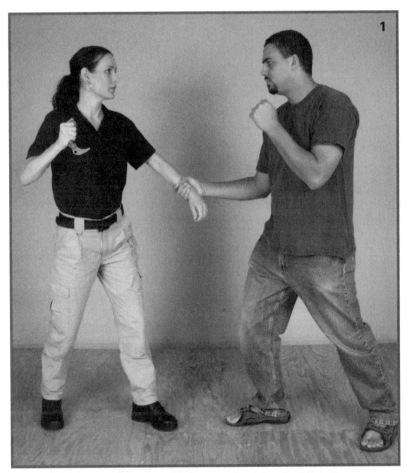

Attack initiates from the left side resulting in a left wrist grab immobilizing the defender.

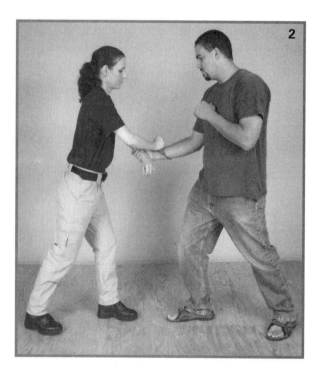

Defender immediately deploys curved blade and delivers distraction to soft target on attacker's wrist while he's still holding on.

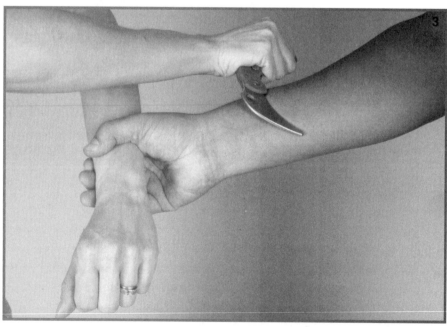

Close up shot of safety mount, blade angle and hand position.

Frontal Attack—Collar Grab Escape Sequence

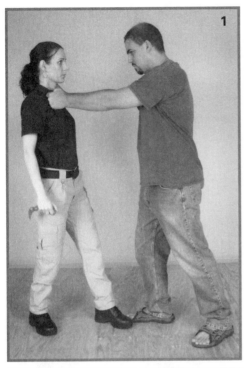

Attacker initiates a frontal assault resulting in a collar grab immobilizing defender.

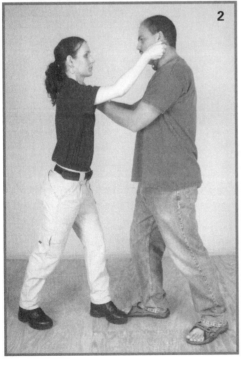

Defender immediately deploys curved blade and delivers distraction to soft target on attacker's throat while he's still holding on. Please keep in mind that this is a LIFE OR DEATH scenario where it is the perception of the defender that she is in immediate danger of loss of life or limb and that the attacker possesses the means, intent and ability to do so. If this were not the case, the defender could just as easily target the nose or hook the mouth or attacker's face.

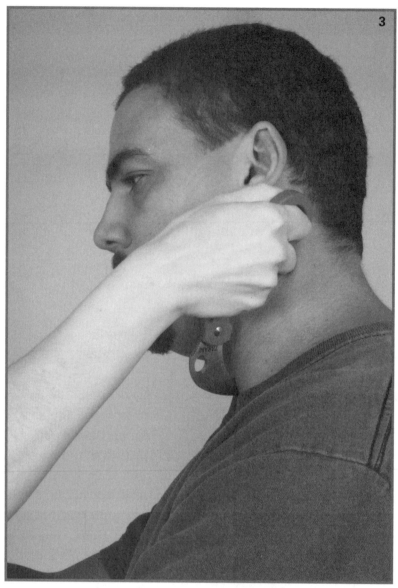

Close up shot of safety mount, blade angle and hand position.

Rear Attack—Double Arm Grab Escape Sequence

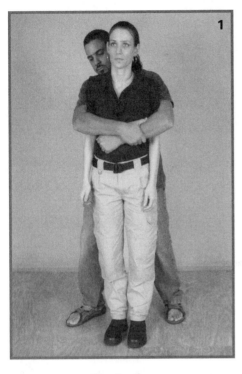

Attack initiates from behind resulting in a double arm grab immobilizing the defender.

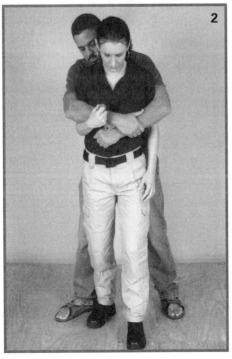

Defender immediately deploys curved blade and delivers distraction to soft target on attacker's wrist while he's still holding on.

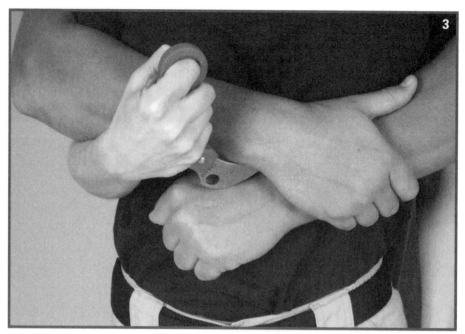

Close up shot of safety mount, blade angle and hand position.

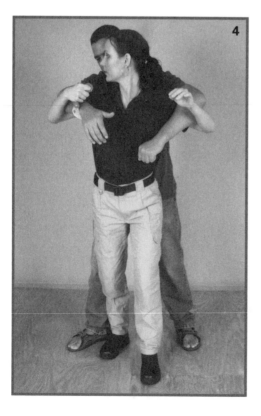

Lifting both elbows straight up while maintaining blade position on attacker's arm, the defender begins to turn and face the threat.

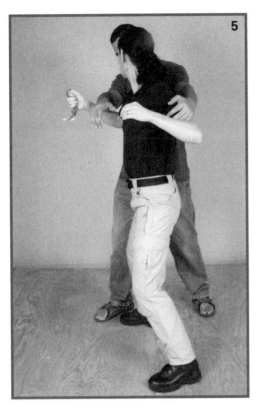

By simply changing her foot position she instantly gains a stable fighting platform, moves to a solid defensive posture and is able to turn and face her threat with blade at the ready.

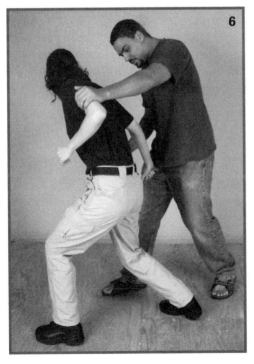

Still unwilling to give up, the attacker attempts to grab the defender a second time which initiates a secondary response of distraction to the groin area thereby releasing his grip and allowing her to move away from the threat area.

Rear Attack—Tight Hair Grab Escape Sequence

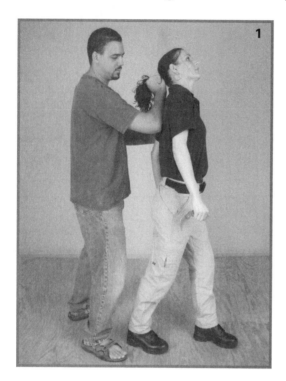

Attack initiates from the rear resulting in a tight hair grab immobilizing the defender.

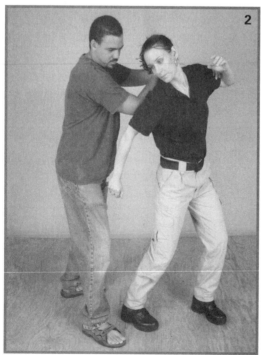

Defender immediately deploys curved blade and delivers distraction to soft target at attacker's groin while he's still holding on and simultaneously turning to face the threat.

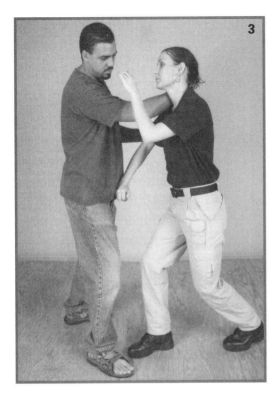

While delivering multiple strikes to the groin area (which brings the attacker's head downward) defender, while gaining a stable fighting platform and squarely facing her threat, moves to apply secondary distraction to the eyes utilizing the fingers of her other hand.

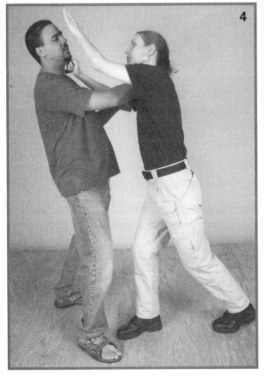

Delivery of secondary distraction to the eyes buys her the time to reposition the blade on a secondary highline target (attacker's face).

Ground Attack—Top Mounted Position Escape Sequence

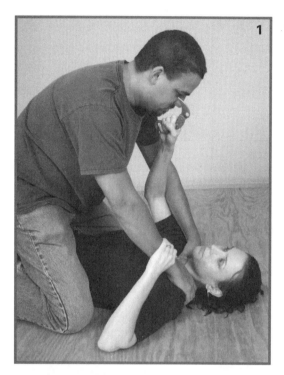

Attack initiates from the ground resulting in a top mount and double hand throat grab immobilizing the defender. Given the obvious suggestive position, the defender immediately deploys her curved blade and applies a distraction to the attacker's face.

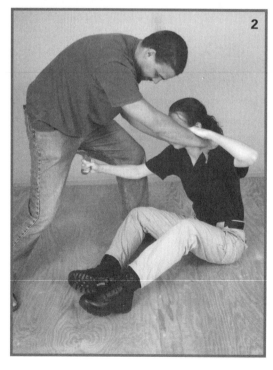

The distraction works enough to cause the attacker to back away a little which creates space. However, he maintains his death grip on her throat. Still immobilized and in bad position on the ground, the defender applies a secondary distraction to the attacker's low-line soft target area (groin).

Ground Attack—Side Mounted Position Escape Sequence

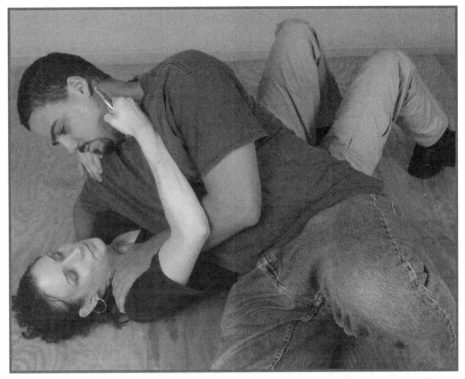

Attack initiates from the ground resulting in a side mount and double hand throat grab immobilizing the defender. Given the obvious suggestive position, the defender immediately deploys her curved blade and applies a distraction to the attacker's face.

Although defender attempts to deliver distractions to attacker's face, he continues to hold on and as he's bigger and stronger and she starts to pass out from his choking grip, she has no other option but to utilize the blade for a secondary distraction.

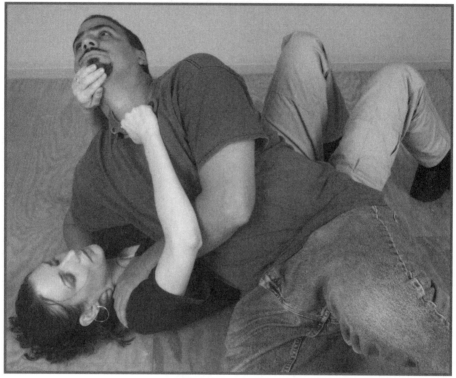

Attacker fails to relinquish his death grip on her throat, on the verge of losing consciousness she transitions from less-than-lethal distraction application to application of the blade directly on a lethal soft target. Notice that she is also utilizing her free hand in order to facilitate escape.

Frontal Attack—Seated Position Escape Sequence

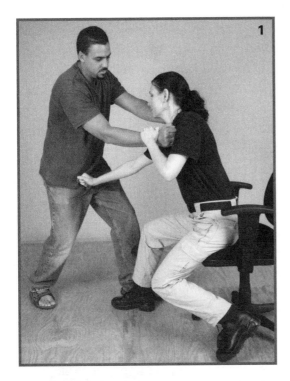

Attack is initiated from the front resulting in a collar grab immobilizing the defender in her seat. Defender immediately deploys curved blade and delivers distraction to soft target at nearest available soft target area (attacker's groin) while he's still holding on. Notice that she has gained a stable fighting platform, has faced her threat and in addition to the blade is utilizing her free hand to assist in her escape.

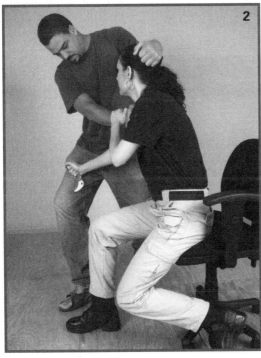

Continuing to face her threat and simultaneously moving from seated position, the attacker fails to remove his deadly grip. The defender, in fear for her life, changes the position of the blade from application to a non-lethal soft target to application of the blade to a potentially lethal soft target.

Practical Application

Unfortunately, in our modern era, an increase in physical violence against humans remains a permanent part of our "civilized" society. Albeit a most unwanted element it is nonetheless undeniable and looms as a pervasive threat to all who choose to move freely through our modern communities.

In order to weave together all previous lessons including technique, concepts and mindset in such a manner as to prepare for personal defense against such attacks to our person, the following section has been provided to allow the reader an overall perspective in putting all the pieces together in the event of practical application.

Frontal attack (grabbing of hair, throat, etc.)—Although any personal attack situation is unwanted, at least from the front you have the most options in regards to awareness and reaction. Assuming flight is not an option due to either lack of distance (and therefore lack of reaction time) or perhaps to protect loved ones, if you do not have access to a firearm, the next best option (if your only remaining option is to stay and fight) is to neutralize the threat. Without any other means of support and to further equalize use of force between you and your attacker (or attackers) accessing and utilizing the curved blade may be your only remaining survival option.

In this example a confined area of engagement limits our choices to victim or victor. Assuming victor is your decision, deploy your curved blade and defend yourself.

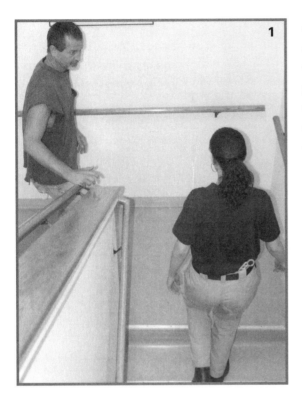

An unfortunate time to be in condition white, the assailant catches us off guard at contact range and takes control of the action/reaction power curve.

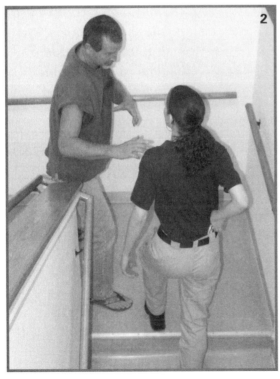

As the attack continues toward true risk of life or limb, having immediate access to the curved blade helps the defender catch up to the power curve.

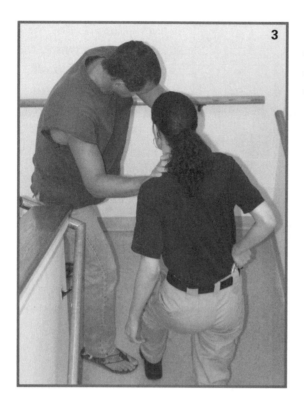

Well within contact range, the assailant makes a life threatening attack at the throat.

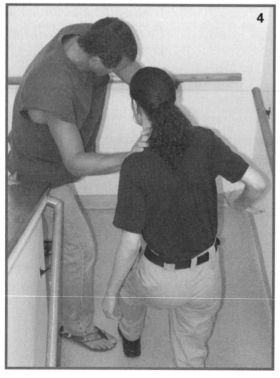

Immediate access to the curved blade allows it to be deployed in a time efficient manner in order to mount a viable defense.

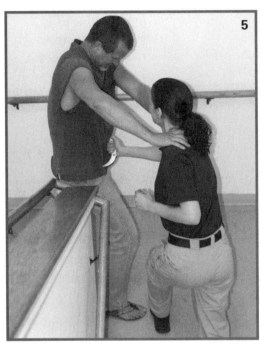

With the assailant's hands still in attack position, a quick soft target strike to the attacker's midsection may cause minor discomfort and place you in control of the power curve. In the heat of interpersonal combat, you have been physically attacked by another human being or possibly even multiple attackers. The only viable response in this ugly situation is to match aggression with aggression—fight fire with fire. Violence of action is the only appropriate response at this critical stage of attack.

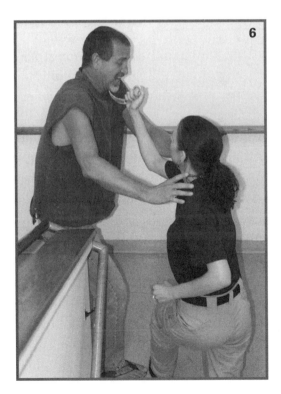

Combination striking with the curved blade allows for maximum effectiveness in defending yourself against violent personal attack.

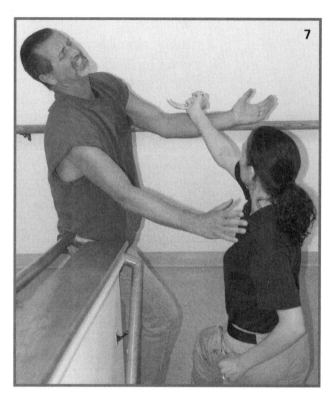

The second strike broke the assailant's hands free. This provides you maximum mobility as well as the ability to continue defending yourself while moving to a position of safety away from the attacker.

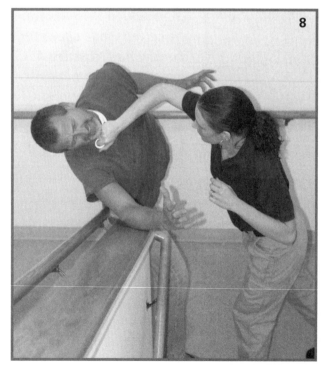

Continuing the combination strike, an additional distraction applied to a soft target against the threat will increase your odds on a successful departure.

Whenever attacked from any direction but head on, it is critical to turn and face the threat as quickly as possible. As covered in previous chapters, this allows you maximum fight or flight options. In this example, the assailant attacks from the left. First and optimal response is to gain immediate distance and run away but in this worse case scenario such an immediate escape is not possible which leaves you with no other option but to engage the threat. Again, deployment of the curved blade may be your only remaining option.

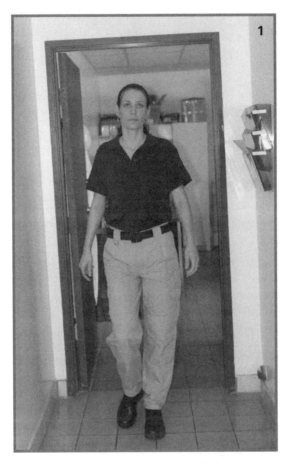

In this example, the attack comes from the left side. Immediately turn to face the threat. If escape is not an option, you can always try and scream and bite and continue to struggle with an opponent who already has the upper hand of surprise attack and superior position. However, deploying your curved blade can equalize use-of-force options and significantly increase your ability to defend yourself.

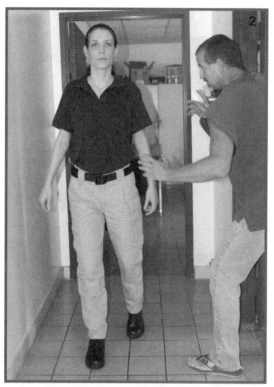

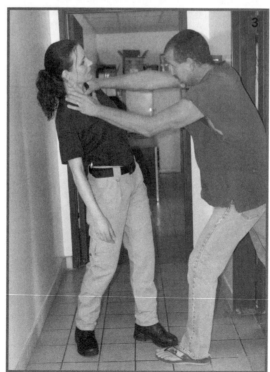

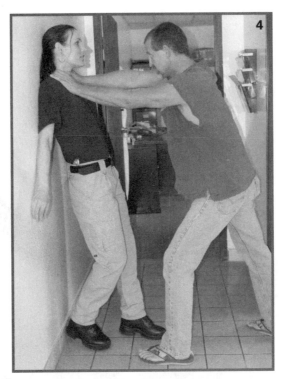

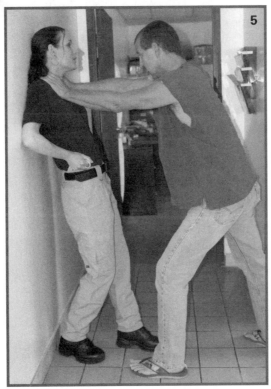

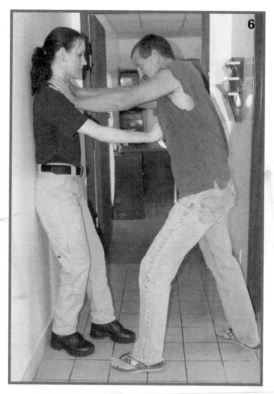

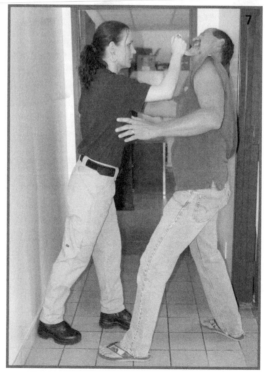

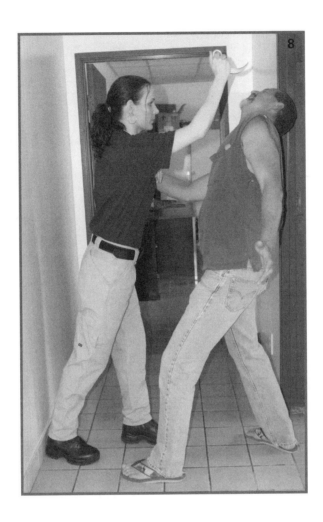

As covered previously, an attack can come from any of 360 degrees around the body—from either a single attacker of multiple attackers. For simplicity of training perspective, we break this down to anterior, posterior, lateral left and lateral right. In this example the attacker has grabbed your knife hand. If access to your curved blade is impeded, strike with your personal weapons (elbow, head butt, knee, kick or even bite or punch the groin or throat) as a distraction in order to loosen his grip which will either allow you to run or, if needed (i.e., if certain risk of loss of life or limb is present), to access your curved blade. One or all of the above responses to such close-quarter violence may significantly decrease your threat to life and severe bodily injury.

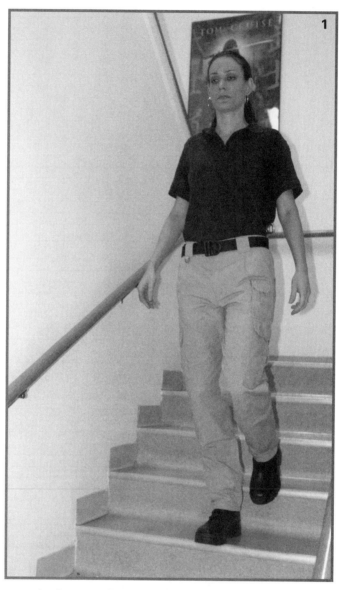

In this example the attack comes from the right, but the curved blade is still accessible to your left hand. Deploy left-handed and acquire available, soft targets. If necessary, application of distractions may be applied to soft targets in such a manner as to fee yourself from the next stage of the attack and move to a position of safety.

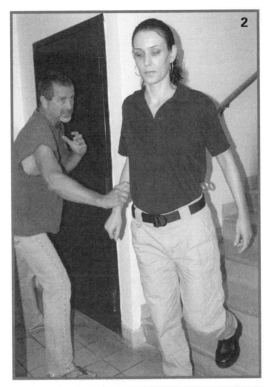

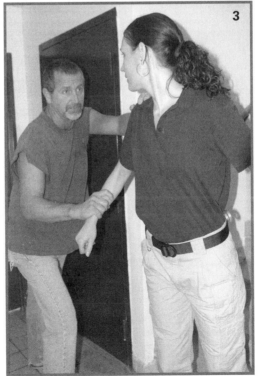

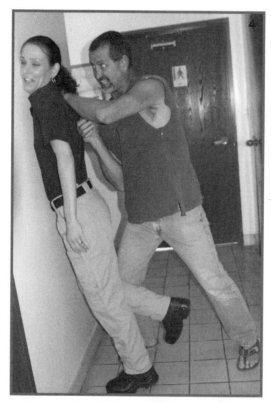

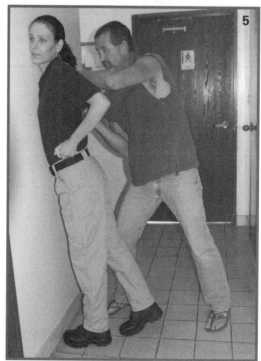

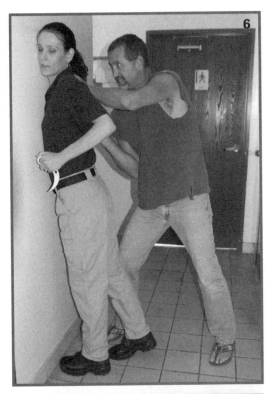

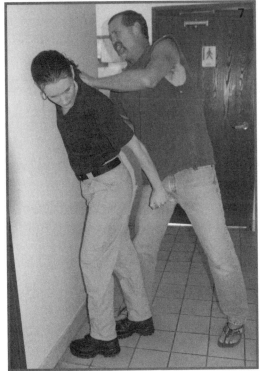

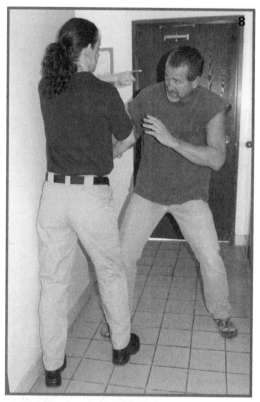

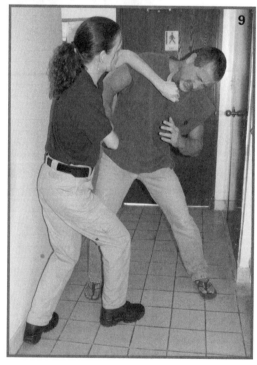

Of all the standing attacks, the attack from the rear is the most serious. You have limited or no visual awareness of the attack and your personal weaponry is extremely limited since it works better face to face. This is very serious business; we're talking murder, rape, all of the above, maybe even the abduction of your child. You need to get your war face on—get your mind into the fight, have a solid plan, immediately turn and face the threat directly by any means possible.

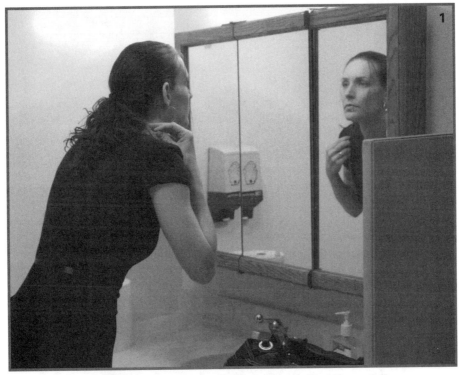

After being attacked from the rear, utilization of the curved blade assists in turning to face the threat as well as effectively defending oneself from the attack.

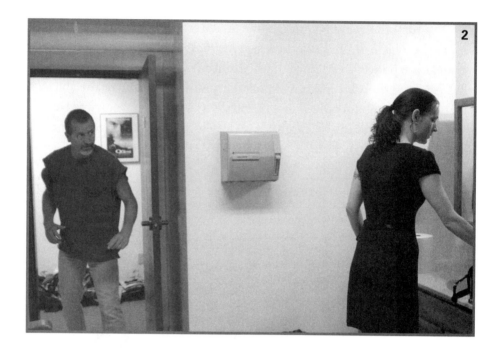

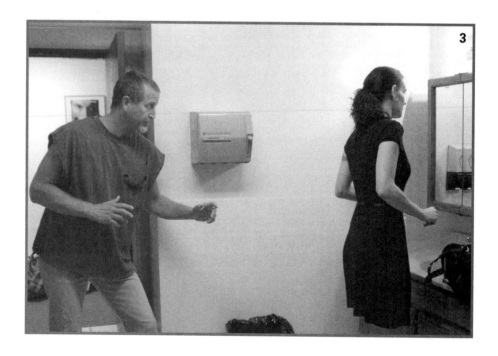

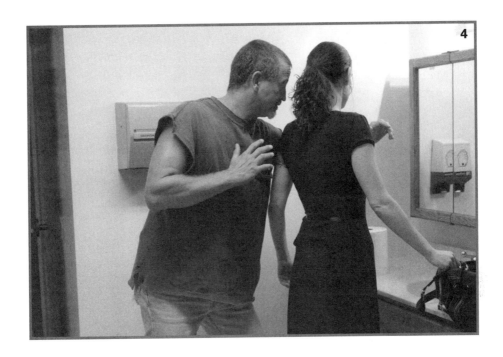

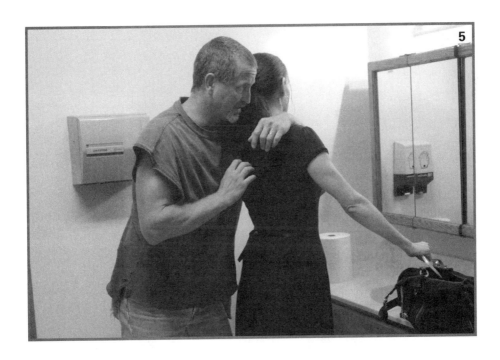

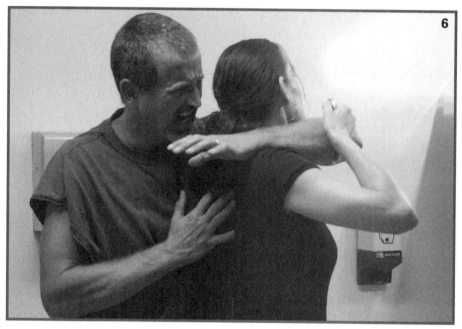

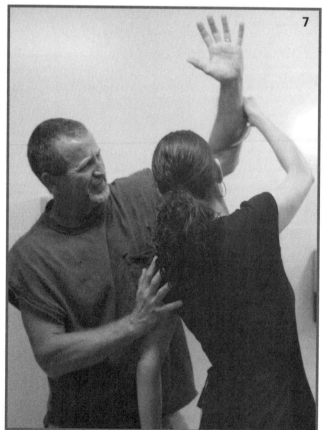

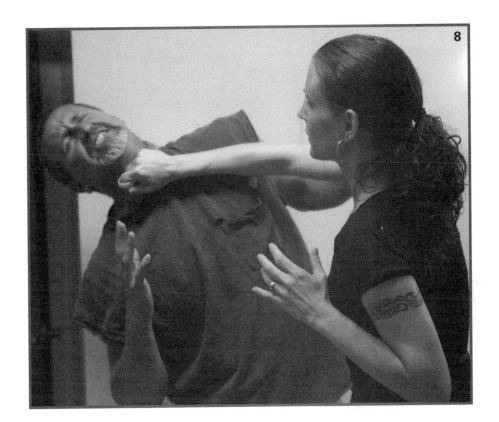

Busy rummaging through the back of your car is another frequent, real life moment of lack of awareness and can easily lead to an attack from the rear.

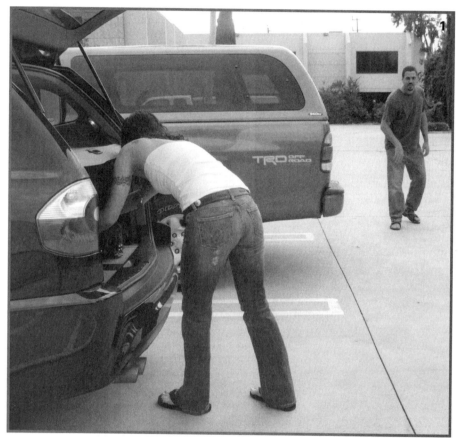

Distracted by narrow focus of attention to her immediate environment, an attack initiates from the rear. Regardless of position of attack, it is essential to turn and face the threat as quickly as possible in order to best defend yourself.

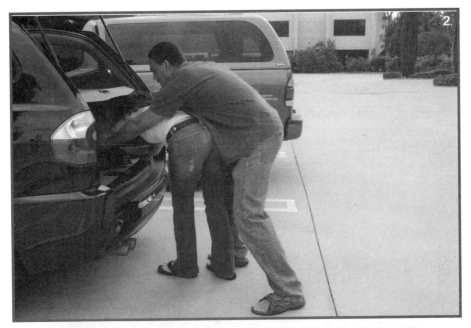

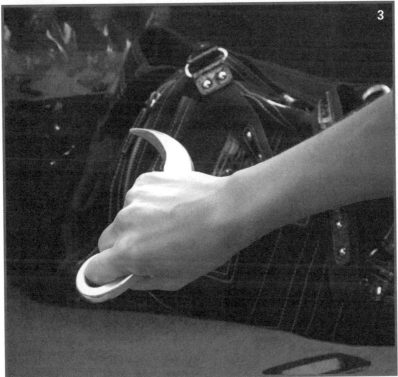

Fortunately for the would-be victim immediate access to her curved blade provides an optimal solution.

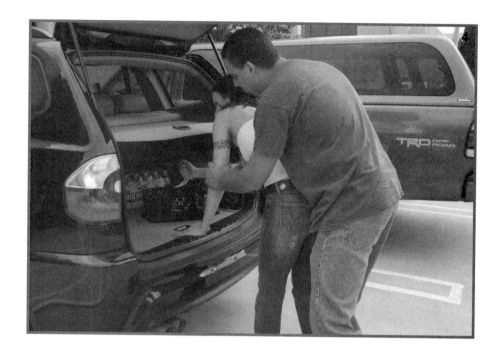

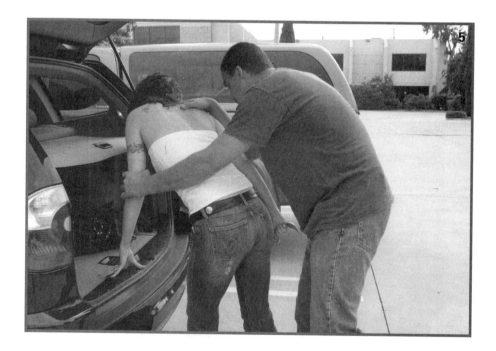

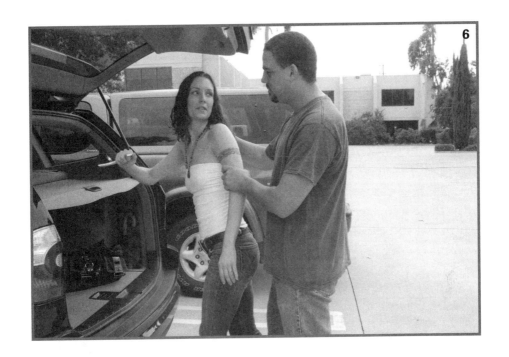

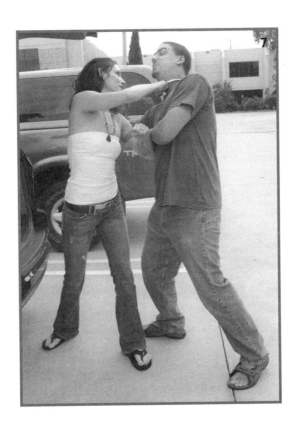

Another unfortunate, but realistic, position to be operationally ready to defend yourself from is the seated position. These include but are not limited to being seated in your car, perhaps at your desk at work, or even out to dinner at a restaurant.

In these examples an unexpected attack comes while seated in the car with the door open and closed. Having your curved blade always accessible is the best way to insure deploying it in a proper and timely manner. When violence comes to you, you must return violence, immediately and effectively. It is a personal choice between victim or victor, which will you choose? Since you're reading this book, we will assume victor is your decision.

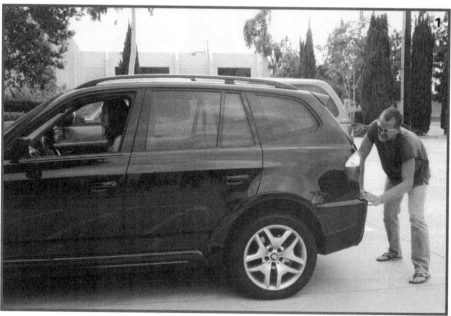

In this particular scenario, note that the trained defender keeps her wits about her in immediately facing the threat and gaining as stable a fighting platform as possible to deliver distractions to her attacker. Her intention is to break free from the attack and remain mobile and not a victim.

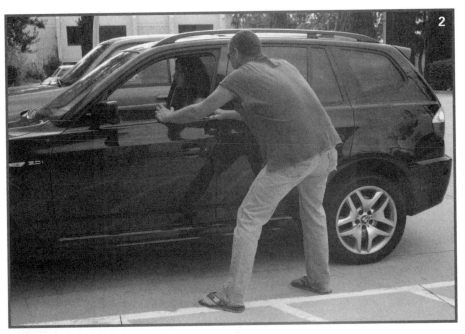

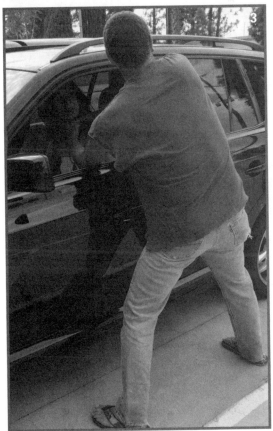

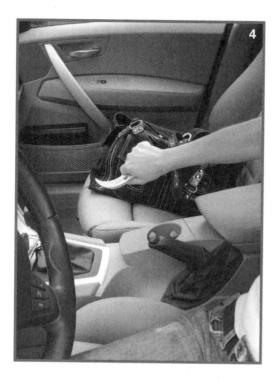

Immediate access to your curved blade is the best way to deploy in a quick and timely manner.

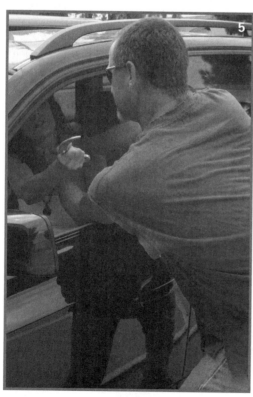

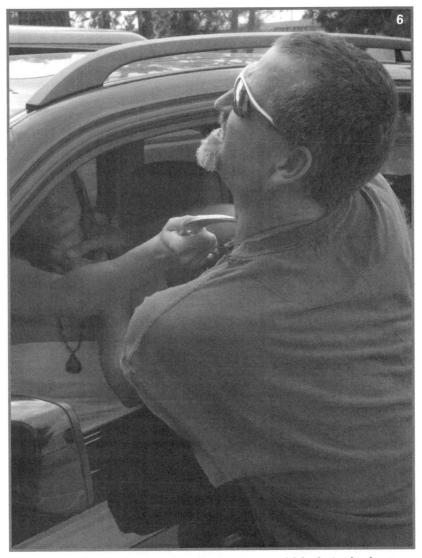

Having immediate access to your curved blade is the best way to deploy in a quick and timely manner. Regardless of your physical position whether standing or seated, if you find yourself in a position of compromise where violence of action is being directed at you, your only two choices are to remain on the receiving end and accept the inevitable consequences or to respond with equal and opposite violence of action to free yourself from the threat of severe and permanent injury or death.

How many times have you gotten out of your car with the phone to your ear or twelve things in your hands or thinking about that jerk who took your parking space? With your environmental awareness dangerously lowered the attacker is able to approach unnoticed and attacks while the car door is open. Even if you are caught behind the power curve with your awareness lowered, the same rules apply: be prepared both physically and mentally to respond. Have your curved blade accessible and be prepared to meet violence with violence.

Fighting from inside a vehicle is certainly less than optimal, however, the same rules of engagement apply: turn and face your attacker, utilize soft target distractions and work yourself as quickly as possible to become mobile and place distance between yourself and the threat.

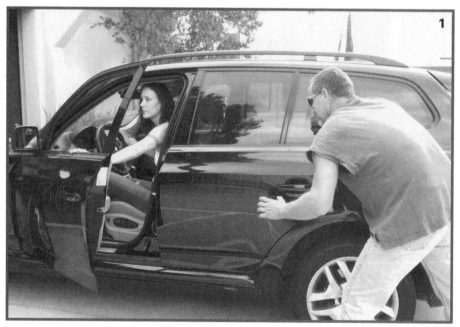

Surprised with the car door open, your options to ensure personal safety are truly limited. In fact you are trying to defend yourself in an extremely confined area of operation. Your attacker is on sure footing and in a far more stable fighting platform with both mobility and accessibility on his side.

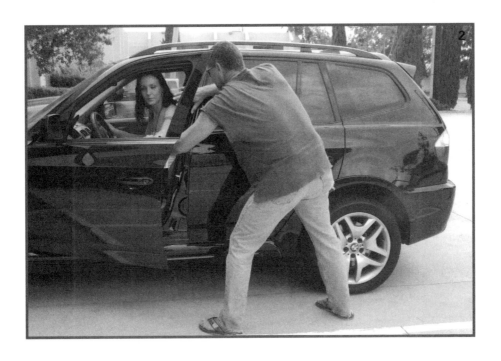

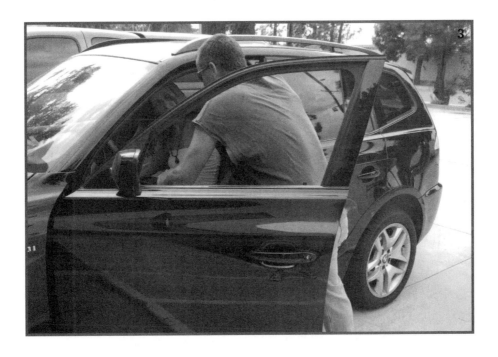

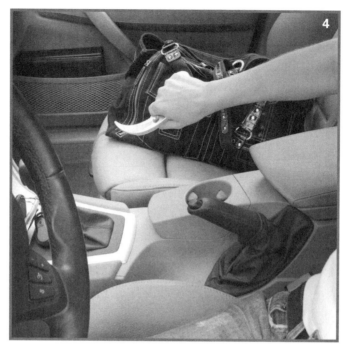

Again, it can be seen in this example that immediate access to your curved blade is the best way to deploy in a quick and timely manner.

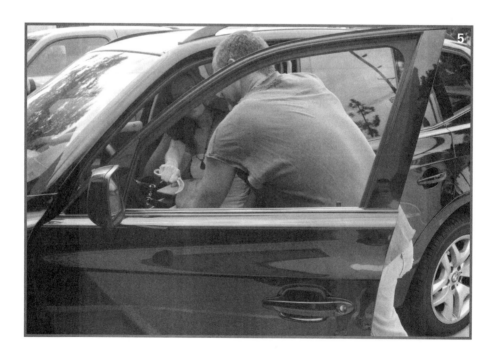

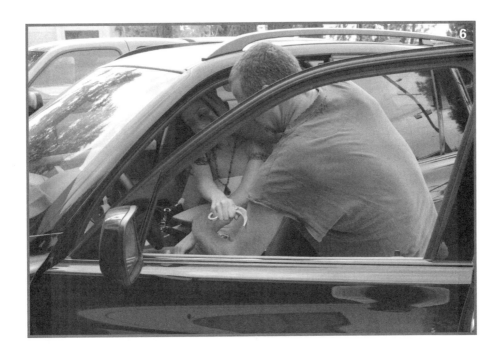

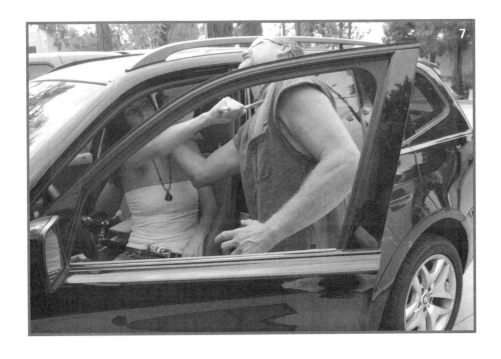

Similar to being seated in the car, at work in the office provides a daily location where the presumption of personal safety lowers your awareness and makes it easier to be caught off guard by an attack. Once again it is imperative to face the threat, and if absolutely necessary, utilize your training and curved blade to defend yourself.

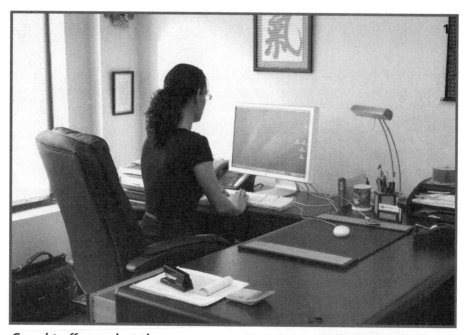

Caught off guard at the workplace. In this series of photos can you identify each of the actions executed by the defender as described in detail in previous chapters? If so, what are they and were they properly executed?

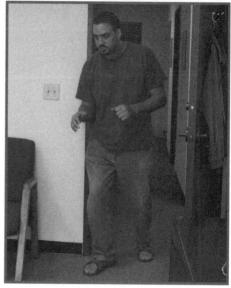

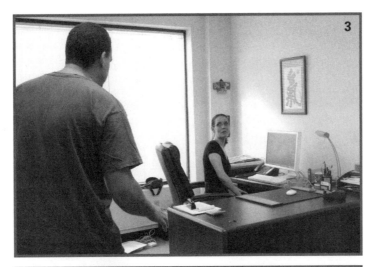

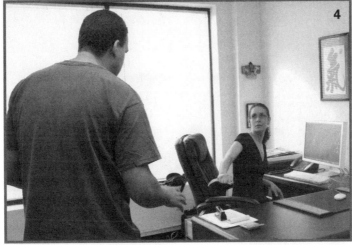

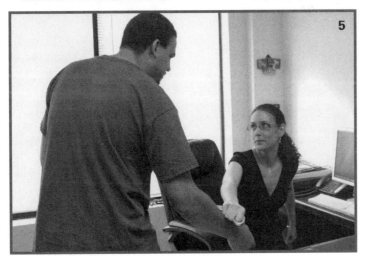

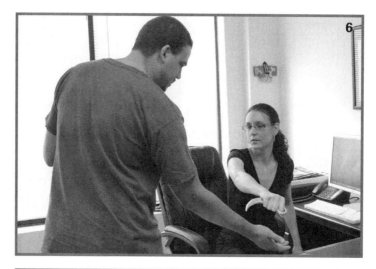

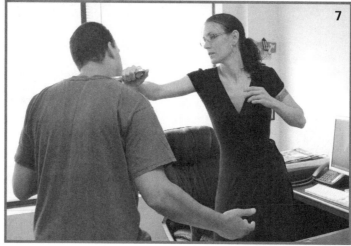

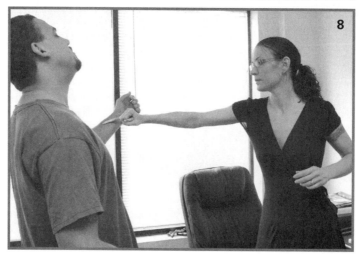

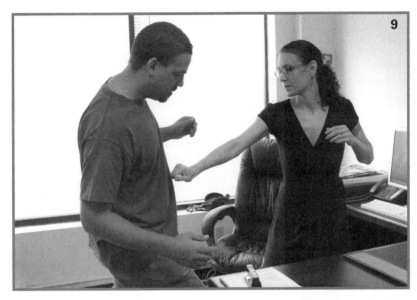

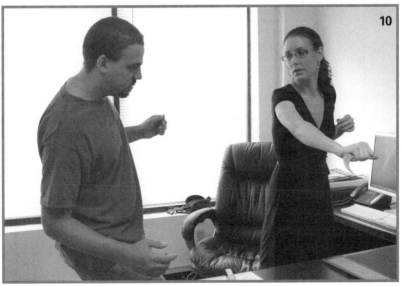

Making a bad situation worse, this example displays being caught off guard, from behind, while seated, and the bad guy gets a handful of hair in an effort to control the fight. Once again, the rules of engagement apply—do whatever it takes to immediately turn and face the threat and applying violence of action to defend yourself against making a bad situation worse.

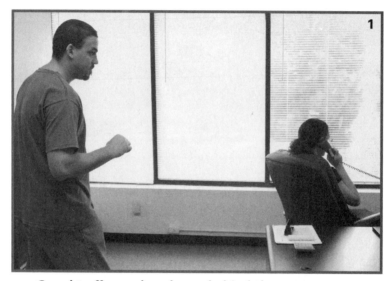

Caught off guard and way behind the power curve,
it is essential to turn and face the threat
and aggressively defend yourself.

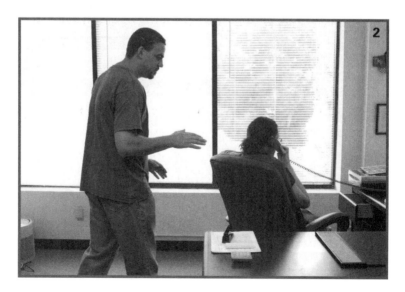

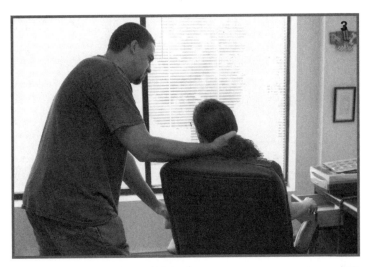

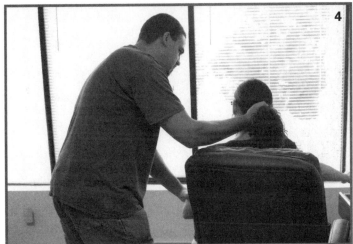

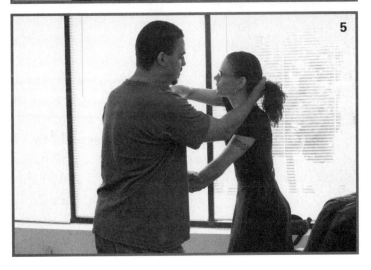

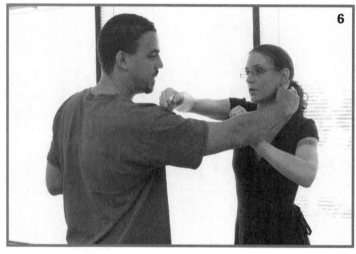

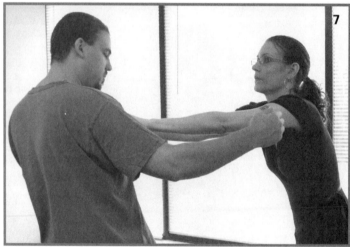

Ground Fighting

One of the most difficult places to defend yourself from is the ground. Whether you're seated on the ground with an attacker closing the distance or you've already been knocked completely on your back with an attacker on top of you, the ground is no place to stay and play. Quickly deploying your curved blade will help equalize your overall position in the fight by shifting use-of-force in your favor in order to survive the attack.

The following examples show a few of the real life situations that you might find yourself fighting from.

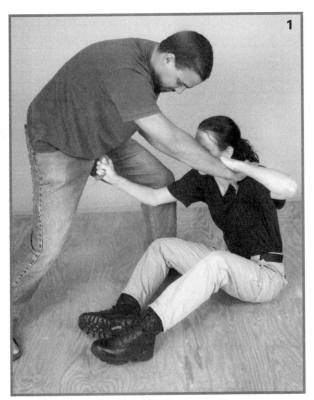

Being seated while your attacker is standing is a very dangerous position from which to be forced to defend yourself. Notice how the curved blade is equally effective in both the standard and reverse grip.

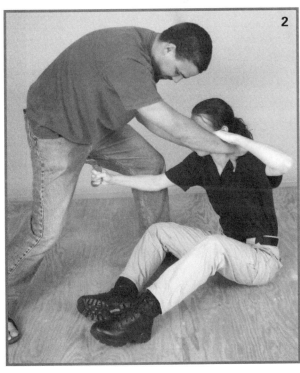

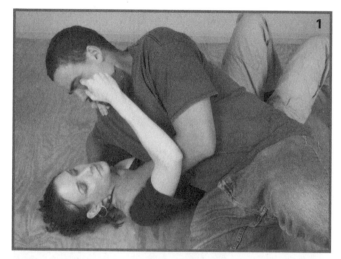

Worse than being seated as now his body weight is on you and the fight is even tougher from the bottom, the curved blade once again works equally well for self defense in either standard grip or reverse grip.

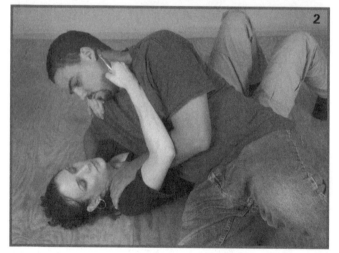

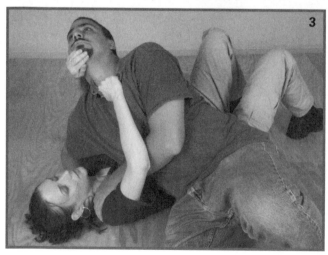

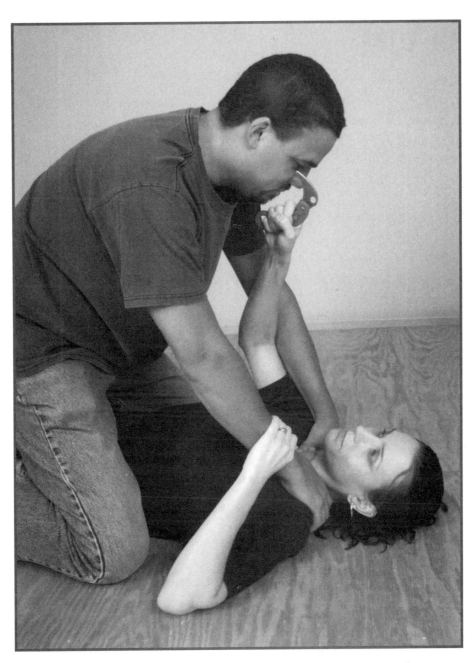

*It doesn't get much worse than this, a bad guy seated
on top in a dominant position. However, the curved blade can
quickly turn victim into victor, even from such a terrible position.*

CONCLUSION

Having been deeply involved in martial arts my entire life and as a full time professional hard-skills instructor providing training services for numerous law enforcement, military and federal agencies since the mid-1990s, I've been fortunate to have met some very squared-away operators over the decades that I deeply respect. Although each of them maintain a continued state of operational readiness, not of one of them goes out looking for a fight. That's because the more you know about fighting, the more you understand its consequences and only do so when there is no other choice. The only time there is no choice is when it is a clear case of defending the life and limb of yourself or your loved ones.

It is my sincere hope there never comes a time that you have to deploy your curved blade for anything other than to open your snail mail, open a Christmas present, or cut a loose thread, but the fact is that we live in violent times and if we have any sense of the future, we know it may get more violent with each passing year. With that understanding of our world, it is better to be prepared than not.

Be ready to go from victim to victor without a conscious thought. The mindset (combative concepts) and personal safety techniques contained herein are simple, gross motor movements that have been battle-proven and can save your life should a deadly threat present itself. Like a good buddy of mine (he's a "former" US Marine) used to say, "Hope for the best, prepare for the worst."

Again, I hope you may never need to use these personal safety skills, but if so, at least you'll have them at the ready.

Stay safe and stay trained,
Steve Tarani
July 2007